# *The complete guide to food for sports performance*

A guide to peak nutrition for *your* sport

**Dr Louise Burke**
*with* Michael McCoy

ALLEN & UNWIN

For my family,
and for my best friend

First published 1992
Allen & Unwin Pty Ltd
9 Atchison Street, St Leonards, NSW 2065 Australia

National Library of Australia
Cataloguing-in-Publication entry:

Burke, Louise.
  The complete guide to food for sports performance.

  Bibliography.
  Includes index.
  ISBN 1 86373 073 7.

  1. Athletes—Nutrition.  I. McCoy, Michael.  II. Title.

613.711

Set in 10.5/11.5 pt Cheltenham, Linotron 300
by Graphicraft Typesetters Ltd, Hong Kong
Printed by Australian Print Group, Maryborough, Vic.

10 9 8 7 6 5 4

# The complete guide to food for sports performance

**WITHDRAWN**

# Forewords

What I eat has always been important to me. I like to think that I was a little ahead of my time in the sports world, not just in realising the connection between nutrition and sports performance, but in putting this into practice in my daily life. During my athletic career, I have seen sports nutrition develop greatly, both in terms of the specialised knowledge now on offer, and the interest generated amongst athletes.

As Director of the Australian Institute of Sport, I am in daily contact with athletes from a variety of sports and can see great differences in the demands and lifestyles of their athletic commitments. It is clear that the time has come to address the special needs of each group individually. *The Complete Guide to Food for Sports Performance* provides a leap forward in this direction. As well as providing an up-to-date review of sports nutrition theory, this book looks at nutrition from inside the athlete's world. A range of sports including swimming, distance running and gymnastics have been examined with detail and insight, raising nutritional issues that can be applied to many other sports as well. The practical advice will be appreciated by athletes of all levels, and provides an important bridge between ideas and action. Any athlete who has had to travel overseas, to eat out in a restaurant with friends, or to carbohydrate load before an event will know that choosing food well is often a challenge.

*The Complete Guide to Food for Sports Performance* is a welcome addition to an athlete's library.

Robert de Castella
Director of the Australian Institute of Sport

It is a great honour to be invited to write a foreword to a text that will go a long way toward reducing one of the many risk factors associated with elite athletic performance.

I have no great knowledge in the areas of nutrition and diet, and as a coach, I am convinced that athletes and coaches do not sufficiently use the expertise and knowledge of those around them with this training.

The author of this book has this knowledge, has used it herself as a triathlete, and is now endeavouring to categorise all sports so that other athletes can get the most benefit from it.

Travelling to swim meets and training camps both in Australia and overseas has given Dr Burke a sound 'hands-on' understanding of how individual athletes think and work. Her advice to team members under my control in both individual and group situations has made a major contribution in giving athletes focus in the correct areas, and the rationale and incentive to keep that focus.

Years ago, even though I held world records, this sort of information would certainly have enhanced my performance as a competitor. We were then instructed not to drink fluids at all on competition days—dehydration was not considered at all; the rationale was that with no fluid intake you would be lighter and not have so much weight to drag through the water. What this did to our metabolism is anyone's guess!

I would have swum every major meet having eaten steak, eggs and chips, believing I needed protein to build muscle. Of course, now we know that if you don't have the muscle by race day, all the protein in the world eaten on that day will not help. Furthermore, I cannot recall the word 'carbohydrate' ever being mentioned.

There are few issues more clouded by misinformation on diet and its effects than athletic performance. Millions of dollars are spent by athletes each year in the hope that some fad diet—rarely based on sound nutritional requirements for the sport followed—or the diet followed by the current champion, will be the easy way.

There is no easy way—in this day and age, we must seek out and respect those who have proven knowledge, and then use it to our best advantage and to help us keep focused.

The task of athletes and coaches today is to eliminate any risk factors that detract from performance, and to maximise potential. This book is a very sound and sincere effort to give you the opportunity to reach your goals.

Terry Gathercole AM
Senior Coach, Australian Institute of Sport
Swimming Coach of the Year 1991

# Contents

# Useful hints and checklists

# Tables

# Figures

# Acknowledgements

Many athletes, coaches and sports scientists provided the inspiration and information for this book. Thank you to all whose who participated in the project, particularly those from the Australian Institute of Sport (AIS). Special greetings go to my great friend and colleague, Vicki, to Rod, and to my muffin-powered swimming team and their wonderful coach.

This book would not have been possible without Mike McCoy, who helped with the research on individual sports, and without all those who proofread and commented on the chapters. None were more patient and dedicated to this task than David Pyne—I thank him for this and for helping to compile data on the physical characteristics of elite athletes.

The heights, weights and skinfold data were kindly supplied by the Department of Physiology and Applied Nutrition and were collected from national and international level athletes using the methods described in Chapter 3. A 'typical physique' was calculated only for sports where sufficient numbers of athletes have been tested, with 'typical' being represented by the mean ± one standard deviation of group values.

# Introduction

Interest in the connection between diet and sports performance is not new. The Ancient Greek Olympians were reported to have eaten special foods to gain strength and endurance. However, until quite recently, sports nutrition has followed a fairly unsophisticated approach. The major focus has been on competition (what should I eat before my event?) where the athlete has treated food almost like a magic wand (if I can eat the right foods then I will be sure to go out and win).

However the last ten years has seen an enormous change in the interest and understanding of optimal nutrition for athletes. Sports scientists have worked hard to unravel many of the mysteries of exercise performance, and we can now identify the special nutritional needs and concerns of athletes arising from their commitment to daily training. In the competition setting, by understanding the physiology of specific sports events, we can pinpoint many of the nutritional and metabolic factors that limit performance—and then find ways to reduce their effect.

The time has come not only to treat each athlete's diet scientifically, but to recognise its individuality. It is no longer sufficient to treat 'the athlete' as a single person: weightlifters, footballers, gymnasts and marathon runners all have their own specific nutrition interests and requirements, arising from their particular training and competition programs. *The Complete Guide to Food for Sports Performance* presents an up-to-date summary of nutrition for athletes—transforming science in practice and taking a look inside the special nutritional needs and lifestyles of various sports.

# I Principles of sports nutrition

# 1 Training nutrition: the principles of everyday eating

Although what you eat before a big event may appear important, it is actually your training diet that holds the most potential to influence sports performance. Consider the many hours that you commit to training each year, to prepare yourself for an event that will last only a fraction of this time—perhaps even only seconds or minutes.

Just from the time angle alone, your everyday diet has most opportunity to make an impact on your body. But more importantly, remember that it is training that lifts you to the stage from which you will compete, and that your diet will play an important role in helping you along the pathway to maximum improvement.

Daily training will create special nutritional needs for an athlete, particularly the elite athlete whose training commitment is almost a full-time job. But even recreational sport will create nutritional challenges. And whatever your level of sport, you must meet your nutritional needs if the maximum return from training is to be achieved. Without optimal training nutrition, much of the purpose of your training might be lost. In the worst case of wasted opportunities, dietary problems and deficiencies may directly impair training performance. However, on the positive side, with the right everyday eating plan your commitment to training will be fully rewarded.

So what is the basis of the optimal training diet? There is no perfect combination of foods or single eating plan that will meet the nutritional challenges of every athlete. If you take a quick look at Part II, you will see that nutritional needs and interests vary between sports. And imagine trying to find one meal plan to encompass the food likes and dislikes, not to mention lifestyles, of all athletes! While the focus and details will differ from one athlete to the next, there are certain goals that are common to all sports. The following checklist will rate the quality of your training diet. If you are achieving all these goals with your everyday eating plan, then congratulate yourself for having achieved peak training nutrition.

Obviously, peak training nutrition doesn't just happen by chance.

---

CHECKLIST FOR PEAK TRAINING NUTRITION

- Can you achieve and maintain a desirable level of body weight and body fat for your sport?

- Do you provide your body with all its nutrient needs, remembering that requirements for some nutrients will be increased by a strenuous training program?

- Do you promote recovery between training sessions with practices that will rapidly replace fluid and fuel stores, and allow the body to recover and adapt to the training load?

- Do you think about the future? Do you take into account the nutrition guidelines for long-term good health? (Not only will this affect the quantity and quality of your own life, but you may be a role model for others who admire your sporting achievements.)

- Do you create opportunities in training to try out your competition eating practices (such as the pre-event meal, or eating and drinking during an event)? Practice makes perfect, and identifies many of the problems that could go wrong on the big day.

---

Before you can branch into the special and individual areas of sports nutrition, you must start with a dietary structure based on the common ground shared by all athletes. Once you have these principles in place, you can then fine-tune your eating plan to account for your particular nutritional needs and dietary goals. At each level, by knowing more about what is in food and ways to select and prepare it, you are in control of what you choose to eat. You can choose to meet your dietary challenges in ways that are both enjoyable to you, and complementary to your busy schedule. So let's start with the basic principles.

### 1.1 Enjoying a variety of food

We have a tendency to oversimplify the food we eat—focusing on one or two nutrients it contains such as iron, chotesterol or sugar. We are quick to pin labels on food—for example, we might believe that yoghurt is 'good' for us while chocolate is 'bad'.

In fact, there is no such thing as a 'good' or 'bad' food. Instead, there are good *uses* of a food—if it contributes toward the achievement of your nutritional goals. This depends on what you are trying to achieve and what else you are eating over the day. A chocolate milkshake might be a great afternoon snack for a hungry basketball player with 'hollow legs'. But two milkshakes in a day would blow the kilojoule budget of a tiny gymnast, and at the 30km mark of a marathon, a runner is looking for a different kind of drink.

Taking the 'good' and 'bad' idea one step further, some people think that a 'good diet' is one where all the bad foods have been removed. So they set themselves the task of giving up all the foods they consider 'bad' (often the ones they enjoy the most). Athletes are particularly skilled at this: they are motivated (often obsessively) and good at self-discipline. No pain, no gain—right? It is not unusual to find athletes who 'out-Pritikin' Pritikin, and who eat a very restricted diet in which many foods, and indeed whole food groups have been removed. At best this may bring some mental satisfaction, but at what cost? All the advantages of a varied diet are lost.

The first step in understanding what is at stake is to appreciate how intricate and sophisticated our food really is. Nutrients do not exist in isolation and are not eaten individually. There is more to an orange than vitamin C, and more to meat than protein. As shown in Figure 1.1, food is a complex mixture of hundreds of chemicals (yes,

**Figure 1.1 Food is a complex mixture of chemicals**

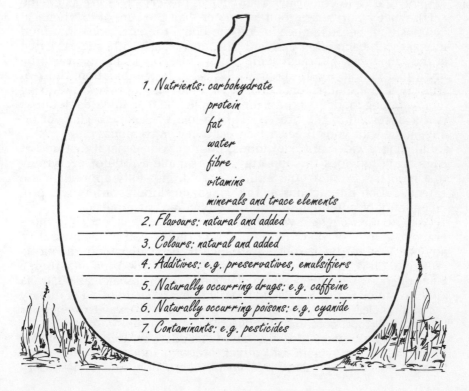

1. *Nutrients: carbohydrate*
   *protein*
   *fat*
   *water*
   *fibre*
   *vitamins*
   *minerals and trace elements*
2. *Flavours: natural and added*
3. *Colours: natural and added*
4. *Additives: e.g. preservatives, emulsifiers*
5. *Naturally occurring drugs: e.g. caffeine*
6. *Naturally occurring poisons: e.g. cyanide*
7. *Contaminants: e.g. pesticides*

---

## HINTS TO ENCOURAGE FOOD VARIETY

- Be prepared to try new foods and new recipes.
- Make the most of foods in season.
- Explore all the varieties of a food. For example, try bread made from different grains other than wheat (rye, multigrain, fruit breads, etc.) and in different forms (sticks, bagels, pita bread etc.).
- Mix and match foods at your meals. Avoid meals made up of just one food type, such as having a fruit-only lunch.
- Think carefully before you banish a food or food group entirely from your diet. Maybe some features do not fit in with your nutritional goals or the dietary principles in this chapter. However, consider what other value the food may have—in particular which other nutrients it could supply. There may be ways to reduce or modify your intake, rather than discard the food totally.

---

carbohydrate and colourings, protein and preservatives are all chemicals). What's more, each food is greater than the sum of its chemical composition, because once inside the body, the chemicals in a food interact with each other and with the chemicals in other foods eaten at the same time. Although some popular diet books have spread the myth that certain foods shouldn't be eaten in combination, the real truth is that the nutritional quality of a meal is improved by mixing and matching foods together. For example, the iron in cereal foods is better absorbed in the presence of vitamin C, making a glass of orange juice with your breakfast cereal a clever combination.

Enjoying a wide variety of foods, both in your general diet and at each meal, provides the opportunity to sample a little of everything that food has to offer. And although we do not fully appreciate the extent of food interactions at this stage, nutritional variety will provide plenty of potential for good combinations at a meal.

From another angle, a varied diet can be viewed as 'eating in moderation'. A little of everything helps to prevent you from overeating any one food, or overexposing yourself to particular food chemicals (whether they be put there by nature or by a food manufacturer). Since the nutritional problems in developed countries such as Australia and the United States are linked mostly to overconsumption of dietary compounds, eating a wide variety of foods is a good way to keep your intake of all food components within healthy levels.

Last, but by no means least, a varied diet offers greater opportunities for flexibility, enjoyment and adventure with food. A major reason that we eat is for pleasure and social interaction, and unnecessary

**Figure 1.2 The food pyramid encourages variety, but gives priority to some foods**

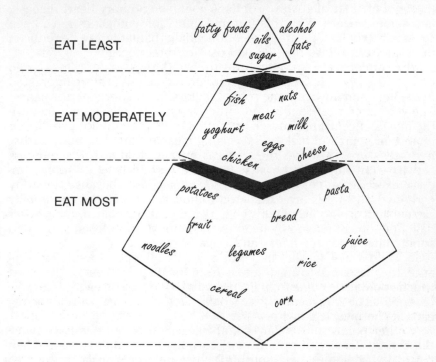

restrictions to your diet will mean an unnecessary sacrifice of this. While optimal training nutrition is about choosing 'a lot of what you need', 'a little of what you fancy' is also part of dietary balance. The food pyramid (Figure 1.2) is a model for the good use of food. Certain foods should be emphasised in your eating program, forming the 'base' of your meals and snacks. However all foods can be part of the scheme—with less nutritious foods taking a small role at the 'tip' of your dietary plan.

## 1.2 Reducing fats and oils

The good news about fats (and oils) in food is that they provide a concentrated source of energy (otherwise known as kilojoules), and make meals tasty, satisfying and rich in texture. They can also supply essential fatty acids and fat soluble vitamins—both important to your health and fitness. The bad news is that too much of a good thing is not necessarily better, and a high fat intake can cause problems. Unfortunately, a high fat diet is second nature to most Australians, with fats and oils providing about 40 per cent of our total energy intake.

Looking at long-term health considerations, there is ample evidence linking a high fat diet with problems such as coronary heart disease, and some cancers. With this in mind, nutrition guidelines have been set for the whole population, recommending that fat intake be reduced by a quarter, to less than 30 per cent of total energy.

While athletes also have their future health to consider (life does go on after the Olympic Games), they are understandably more interested in the here and now, and the role of dietary fat in sports performance. The verdict on this front is that although fats and oils in your diet are the most concentrated source of food energy, they do not provide an important source of fuel for exercising muscles. Instead, body carbohydrate stores provide the critical energy source for strenuous activity—critical firstly because below a certain level of supply, intense exercise cannot be maintained, and secondly because the body carbohydrate stores are exhausted in hours and must be continually replenished from carbohydrate in the diet. Body fat, on the other hand, is in plentiful supply even in the leanest of athletes, and could supply fatty acids for hours and days of exercise.

So while a high-fat diet may not directly influence sports performance, the disservice to an athlete is from the displacement of kilojoules which could have come from carbohydrate foods. The energy from fat contributes heavily to an athlete's daily kilojoule budget without taking care of the muscle's fuel needs.

Another point to consider is that because fats and oils have twice the energy density of protein and carbohydrate (that is, more than twice the kilojoules per mouthful), high-fat foods make it easy to overeat your daily energy requirements. And that means you gain body fat! A lower-fat diet can help to prevent you from gaining excess body fat by making you need more mouthfuls to reach your energy needs. Conversely, when weight loss (loss of body fat) is on the agenda, cutting back fat intake is the most effective way of reducing your kilojoule intake.

Figure 1.3 illustrates the energy situation in food.

So how much fat should an athlete eat? This question is best answered by first determining your daily kilojoule requirements for protein and carbohydrate. The remaining kilojoules can be then filled in  with fat. For most athletes, as for the rest of the community, cutting back fat and oils to less than 30 per cent of total energy intake is a suitable goal. For athletes whose kilojoule needs are in short supply (small eaters and those trying to lose weight), it may be necessary to cut back the fat intake to 12–20 per cent of total energy intake to allow for other nutrient needs. A similar ratio might be suitable for endurance athletes with heavy daily training schedules, to make way for their large requirements for carbohydrate energy.

The important point to remember is that dietary fat should not be left out all together. Some nutrition books (and many athletes) have

**Figure 1.3 What is energy?**

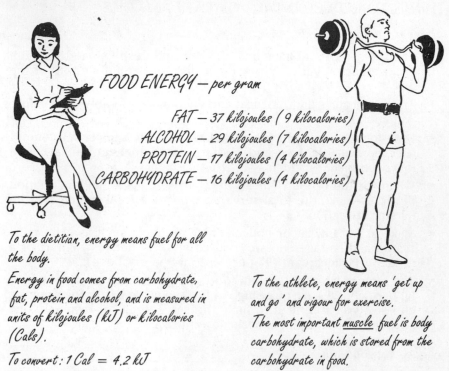

FOOD ENERGY – per gram

FAT – 37 kilojoules ( 9 kilocalories)
ALCOHOL – 29 kilojoules (7 kilocalories)
PROTEIN – 17 kilojoules (4 kilocalories)
CARBOHYDRATE – 16 kilojoules (4 kilocalories)

To the dietitian, energy means fuel for all the body.
Energy in food comes from carbohydrate, fat, protein and alcohol, and is measured in units of kilojoules (kJ) or kilocalories (Cals).
To convert: 1 Cal = 4.2 kJ

To the athlete, energy means 'get up and go' and vigour for exercise.
The most important muscle fuel is body carbohydrate, which is stored from the carbohydrate in food.

tried this approach, attempting to reduce fat to less than than 10 per cent of the diet or even no fat at all. This might sound like good economy, but in real life it is impossible to achieve without sacrificing variety and its benefits. Small amounts of fat are found in many important foods, and fat 'headhunters' will eventually pay for cutting them out of their diets. Stick to the moderate angle: trim the excess and enjoy the valuable.

A last word on the different types of fat in food. There is much that is still being learned about the role of various chemical forms of fat and oils in food—saturated, monounsaturated, polyunsaturated, cholesterol and so on. A good nutrition textbook can fill you in if you want to pursue this further. However, the best advice overall is probably to make up your total fat quota with a little of each type.

## 1.3 Increasing your carbohydrate intake

Carbohydrate foods play a vital role in exercise performance. The critical source of fuel for exercising muscles comes from your body's

# HINTS TO REDUCE INTAKE OF FATS AND OILS

*Protein and dairy foods*

- Choose lean cuts of meat and chicken, and fresh fish and seafood. Choose non-oil varieties of canned fish, or carefully drain off the oil.

- Trim all fat and skin from meat and chicken—preferably even before you cook it.

- Look for new types of processed meats with a lower fat content (92 per cent fat-free and above). Avoid high-fat sausage and luncheon meat products.

- Whatever the protein—meat, fish, chicken, egg or a combination of these—make the total serve *accompany* a meal rather than be its star attraction.

- Make use of low-fat or non-fat dairy products such as skim milk, ricotta and cottage cheese. For desserts, try non-fat yoghurt or a little low-fat icecream (97 per cent fat-free or above).

- The highest-fat dairy protein food is cheese. Even many reduced-fat hard cheeses are quite high in fat, and while better than regular cheeses, you still need to limit the serve size—for example, one slice in a sandwich or a sprinkle on pizza.

*Added fats and oils*

- Become a whizz with non-fat (or minimum fat) cooking methods. Grill, bake on a rack or in foil, microwave, steam, or 'dry fry' with a non-stick frypan or a tiny smear of oil.

- Watch the amount of butter or margarine you add to foods, particularly bread. Use a scrape, or better still, none.

- Use no-oil dressings, low-fat mayonnaises or lemon juice to liven up salads. Avoid butter- and cream-based sauces and gravies. You can often make your own with low-fat ingredients.

- Avoid cream and sour cream—try non-fat plain yoghurt instead.

*Snack foods and take-aways*

- Snack foods such as chips, corn chips and nuts are high in fat—as well as being very 'moreish'. Keep away from the bowl when these foods are served. You can make your own low-fat snacks by popping corn (with minimal oil), or by toasting strips of pita bread to make 'chips' for dips. Raw vegetables can also be chopped into bite-size snacks.

- Take-aways are often high in fat—especially if fried, battered or in pastry. Hopefully they do not make up a big part of your diet. When having take-aways, choose types that are lower in fat, and order a small serve (add other nutritious foods to make up the rest of the meal).

*Processed foods*

- Learn to read labels to estimate the fat content of packaged foods (see Figure 1.4). Try to choose those that are lower in fat—if you can calculate the ratio of fat to total energy in a food, stick to those in which less than 30 per cent of kilojoules come from fats/oils (Figure 1.4 again). There are lower fat substitutes for many foods—e.g. scones or bagels instead of croissants, low-fat icecream instead of icecream or cheesecake.

- It is possible to make reduced-fat versions of cakes, puddings and desserts. You can make your own from 'healthy' recipe books or modify your favourite recipes to reduce the amount of butter, oil, margarine and other high-fat ingredients. There are also a number of commercial brands of these items now appearing on supermarket shelves.

- Enjoy chocolate, chocolate biscuits, pastries and rich cakes as a treat. If you go for quality with the foods that are special to you, you won't mind a smaller quantity.

carbohydrate stores—in the form of blood glucose (a small amount), and glycogen stored in the liver and muscles (larger stores, but still only sufficient for up to 90 minutes of continuous intense exercise). These stores must be continually refilled from the carbohydrate in your diet, and obviously the more you exercise the greater your dietary carbohydrate needs will be.

Currently, carbohydrate provides about 40–45 per cent of the total energy in the Australian diet. For the athlete a minimum target of 50–60 per cent is set, with higher levels again for endurance athletes and those undertaking lengthy daily training sessions. With carbohydrate making such a large contribution to total energy needs, the most important food choices will be those that can supply additional nutrient value. After all, your peak training diet must achieve a number of other goals as well as contribute to muscle glycogen stores.

Traditionally, carbohydrate foods have been classified in terms of the chemical structure of the carbohydrate molecule—being 'simple carbohydrates' of one or two molecules (known as sugars) and 'complex carbohydrates' made up of thousands of molecules (known as

**Figure 1.4 How can you tell the fat content of food?**

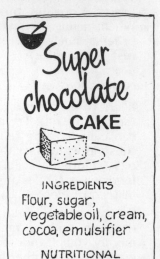

*HINT ONE:* Read the ingredient list on the label. These are listed in descending order:

- If fat is in the 'Top Three', or listed several times by various names, then this food is probably high in fat.
- Fat may be hidden under the following aliases: vegetable fat, vegetable oil, animal fat, shortening, lard, cream, butter, margarine, copha.....

*HINT TWO:* Calculate the fat – energy ratio from nutrition information. It may be on the label, or perhaps you can find it in a 'Kilojoule Counter' or Food Table book.

- Multiply the number of grams of fat in a serve by 37
  Divide by total kilojoules in the same serve
  Multiply by 100
  (For kilocalories, multiply by 9 and divide by Cals)

Example: Super chocolate cake — 50g serve

$$\text{Fat – energy ratio} = \frac{8 \times 37}{795} \, kJ \times 100$$

$$= 37\%$$

- Try to choose foods with less than 30% of energy from fat.

---

starches). However, this classification system tells us nothing about the overall nutritional value of these foods, or even about the way they will behave in the body. You may have heard stories about 'sugars' causing a rapid rise in blood glucose levels (followed by a rapid fall), while complex carbohydrates create a gentle blood glucose curve. This concept is in fact quite inaccurate.

New diabetes research has shown that each carbohydrate-rich food has a unique effect on blood glucose and other body physiology, and this can be quite unconnected to its 'simple' or 'complex' form. A ranking system has been created comparing individual carbohydrate foods according to the rate at which they release glucose into the bloodstream. This system, called the Glycemic Index, may have applications in sport if it can be used to manipulate favourable blood glucose conditions for special purposes—for example, the optimum blood glucose level at the start of exercise, or the optimum level to promote maximum glycogen synthesis after exercise has finished.

However, these ideas require further research and experimentation. For the present, the priority in your everyday training diet is to select 'nutritious' carbohydrate foods which can simultaneously contribute to a number of your dietary goals.

While a system describing the nutritional value of foods will always be arbitrary, we can try to simplify carbohydrate-rich foods into categories of 'nutritious' and 'less nutritious'. 'Nutritious' relates to the content of carbohydrate and other nutrients compared to the total energy content—and most of the time you will be after maximum nutritional value for minimum kilojoules. 'Nutritious' carbohydrate-rich foods can be described as those also providing valuable amounts of vitamins, minerals, protein or fibre for a moderate kilojoule intake. 'Less nutritious' carbohydrate sources include foods that have been processed to remove much of their nutritional value or foods in which fat and sugar add lots of kilojoules and dilute the total nutrient–energy ratio. Figure 1.5 provides example of carbohydrate-rich foods in both categories.

Traditionally, 'simple carbohydrate'-containing foods have been regarded as 'less nutritious' foods, while all 'complex carbohydrate'-rich foods have been considered 'nutritious'. Figure 1.5 shows that this concept is also not true—there are both differences and overlaps between the two ideas. Just as some carbohydrate foods based on 'simple carbohydrates' provide a valuable source of vitamins and fibre (e.g. an orange), there are 'complex carbohydrate' foods that contain far more fat and kilojoules that you bargained for, and little in the way of fibre, vitamins and minerals (e.g. a Danish pastry). There are also carbohydrate-rich foods that contain significant amounts of both 'complex' and 'simple' carbohydrates, thus straddling the traditional classification lines (e.g. cakes).

A good start to the peak training diet is to turn typical Australian eating habits inside-out. Carbohydrate-rich foods should now become the base of all meals and snacks, and amongst these the 'nutritious' carbohydrate-based foods should take pride of place. We will see later that 'less nutritious' carbohydrate-rich foods can also play a role—often being a practical or enjoyable means of consuming carbohydrates. But the first step is to change your attitude and become

*13*

**Figure 1.5  Carbohydrate foods**

| REFINED CARBOHYDRATES | UNREFINED/NUTRITIOUS CARBOHYDRATES | |
|---|---|---|
| • sugar<br>• honey, jam<br>• syrups, toppings<br>• glucose, fructose<br>• soft drinks, cordial, flavoured mineral water<br>• sports drinks, high carbohydrate supplements (carbo-loaders)<br>• sweets, chocolates<br>• high-fat cakes, pastries, biscuits and desserts (high fat and sugar) | • fruit<br>• fruit juice<br>• canned fruit<br>• dried fruit<br>• milk, yoghurt<br>• liquid meals (Sustagen, Exceed Sports Nutrition Supplement etc.)<br>• low-fat cakes, biscuits, desserts (scones, pancakes, special recipes etc.) | SIMPLE CARBOHYDRATES |
| • pastry<br>• chips<br>• crisps, Twisties, etc.<br>• high-fat cakes, pastries, biscuits and desserts | • breads<br>• breakfast cereals<br>• pasta and noodles<br>• rice and other grains<br>• starchy vegetables<br>• legumes<br>• low-fat cakes, biscuits, desserts (scones, pancakes, special recipes) etc.)<br>• dry biscuits and rice cakes | COMPLEX CARBOHYDRATES |

*Carbohydrate foods can be classified according to the chemical form of the carbohydrate — but a better classification system rates the total nutritional value of the food. Note that some foods, such as cakes, contain significant amounts of both simple carbohydrate (sugar) and complex carbohydrate (flour).*

## HINTS TO EMPHASISE NUTRITIOUS CARBOHYDRATE-RICH FOODS IN YOUR DIET

- Be prepared to be different. A typical Western diet is *not* a high carbohydrate diet. You will need to plan ahead, be organised, and on occasions 'stand away from the crowd'. Hopefully however, your high-carbohydrate diet being the blue-print for healthy eating, other people will follow your lead.

- Plan each meal around a carbohydrate food, making it the centre of attention and adding the rest of the meal around it—for example, add filling to a sandwich, sauce to pasta, topping on breakfast cereal. Otherwise, take your traditional meal, cut the protein serve in half and add a generous serve of carbohydrate foods (bread rolls, potatoes, rice, etc.) to fill up more than half the plate.

- Choose breakfast cereals from the low-sugar, high-fibre range. Look out for toasted mueslis—they are high in fat and sugar. Make your own muesli recipe or use the commercial toasted varieties as a sprinkle over other cereals.

- Enjoy the sweetness and variety of fruit at meals and snacks. Fresh is usually the most nutritious form—but make good use of juices and dried, canned and stewed fruits.

- Explore bread in all its forms—pita, bagels, rolls, crumpets, damper and fruit bread to name but a few. Go for thick-sliced loaves, or bread rolls to increase the bread part of the sandwich.

- Cakes, slices and puddings can be high in fat. Scones and pancakes are a great choice—or experiment with reduced-fat recipes for wholemeal cakes, muffins, and wholemeal puddings. Modify your own recipes or find low-fat commercial varieties (e.g. Pritikin style).

- Other low-fat carbohydrate desserts include non-fat fruit yoghurts, and low-fat icecream or ice-desserts. Otherwise, make your own recipes based on fruits.

- Become versatile with pastas and noodles in all their shapes and sizes. Eat them plain as a side dish, or add a low-fat sauce and make a meal. Rice can also be used in this way—with main dishes including paella and fried rice (dry-fried of course).

- Try legumes (kidney beans, lentils, chick peas, etc.) in pasta sauces and casseroles to replace some or all of the meat, fish or chicken. Make a hearty soup or bean salad a meal in itself.

- Make the most of starchy vegetables—potatoes, corn, peas, etc. Baked potatoes and corn on the cob can pep up a meal, and stuffed potatoes make a delicious main meal.
- Note that other vegetables, particularly salad vegetables, are good sources of fibre as well as some vitamins and minerals. However, they are not good sources of carbohydrate by themselves and should be eaten with other carbohydrate foods at the meal.
- Low fat 'carbo shakes' can be made with skim milk, fruit and ice cubes. Low fat icecream and non-fat yoghurt are optional extras for a creamy drink.
- Be adventurous with your cooking. Vegetarian and healthy recipe books can provide clever ways of making cereals, grains and vegetables the focus of a meal.

creative with the foods that we have traditionally made the afterthought in our eating habits. You'll know you have it right when you start thinking 'maybe I'll have a rice dish or stuffed potatoes for tea' rather than 'I'll roast a leg of lamb or defrost some steak from the freezer'.

A good reason for choosing nutritious carbohydrate foods is that they often provide a good source of fibre—a nutrient forgotten until recently. Unfortunately, sprinkling bran on your cornflakes, or eating oatbran muffins by the truckload does not do justice to the fibre story.

Fibre is not one substance, but rather a family of compounds that exert different effects on the metabolism of food in the body. This includes aiding digestion, regulating blood glucose and blood cholesterol levels, and reducing the risk of some cancers.

Fibre is found in plant and vegetable foods—or more precisely, fibre occurs *naturally* in these foods. Quite often the processing of food removes the fibre—not just in the food factory, but in the restaurant or in your kitchen. It is not uncommon for people to eat processed food, minus its fibre, and then buy bran to sprinkle onto other dishes. But the best guideline is to eat fibre as it would naturally be found in the variety of foods that you eat. This will ensure that you get a mixture of the fibre types and that quantity of fibre varies in ratio with your energy and nutrient intake.

Like anything, too much fibre has its disadvantages. Fibre adds bulkiness and volume to foods, making the meal more filling. This can be a friend to those with low energy requirements, but can make life difficult for athletes with heavier energy needs. Be guided by a sensible amount and variety of fibre.

And finally to sugar, which also suffers confusing publicity. On the

---

HINTS FOR A HEALTHY FIBRE INTAKE

• On most occasions choose foods with the fibre content left intact by:

— selecting wholegrain breads and breakfast cereals, wholemeal pastas and brown rice

— enjoying some of your fruits and vegetables raw—for example, fresh fruit, salads, crunchy vegetable sticks, fruit salad, whole fruits blended into 'smoothies'. Eat the skins and seeds where appropriate.

— cooking fruit and vegetables lightly, leaving them a little crisp rather than overcooked. Again, leave the skins on where appropriate.

• Cook with wholemeal flour. Start by replacing half the white flour in your recipes with wholemeal. In many cases you may find that 100 per cent wholemeal is the way to go.

• Experiment with vegetarian recipes or ideas. Try legumes and other types of grains and cereals.

• There is probably no need for added fibre, such as unprocessed brans, unless they are part of a whole food recipe.

---

one hand it is labelled 'pure, white and deadly' and blamed for all manner of health problems. On the other, it is hailed as 'a natural part of life', and even an 'energy food' for athletes. Who is telling the truth?

Sugar is the popular name for sucrose, the most commonly occurring simple sugar in the western diet. Of all carbohydrate foods, this is the most refined, being extracted from sugar cane and purified to remove all other compounds, including any other nutrients. In all forms, sugar and related substances such as honey, glucose and fructose provide carbohydrate and kilojoules, and little else.

Medical research now recognises that sugar itself is not the direct cause of disease, apart from its contribution to tooth decay. It is more by association that sugar is related to health problems. Sugar is a compact and delicious form of kilojoules, especially in the form of sugar-coated fats such as chocolate, cake and icecream. And this combination of high kilojoules and fat, minus the fibre, vitamins and minerals is where the potential for overuse and subsequent health disadvantages lie. The current intake of sugar in Australia—almost a kilogram a week, or about 20 per cent of total energy intake—means that sugar is overstating its role in the total dietary picture.

HINTS FOR USING SUGAR WELL

- Look at the total amount of sugar that you eat. Try to keep this to about 10 per cent of your total energy intake.
- When weight loss is desired, take a stronger hand to reduce sugar intake and save the kilojoules for more nutritious carbohydrate foods.
- Enjoy sugar-coated fat foods as a treat. Think of chocolate, icecream, and rich cakes as 'fun' foods rather than 'energy' foods, and give them a special rather than a regular place in your eating plan.
- Use sugar as an addition to your base of nutritious carbohydrate foods—such as a little jam on toast, syrup on pancakes, soft drink with a meal. But, don't let it take over the show.
- Apart from times when a carbohydrate drink is specifically required for your sports performance, stick to water, low-joule drinks and plain mineral water.
- Good ways to cut back the extra sugar are:
  - gradually cut back what you add to your coffee or sprinkle on your breakfast cereal
  - look for 'unsweetened' and 'no-added-sugar' brands
  - experiment with recipes to cut back the added sugar
  - make use of low-joule artificial sweeteners, especially where energy needs are tight. Of course, treat such sweateners with respect—you can overdo the use of these as well.
  - learn to read labels in order to recognise sugar by its other names (sucrose, fructose, corn syrup, glucose, etc.).
- Care for your teeth by eating sugary foods as part of a meal, and try to have your toothbrush around when sticky, sugary foods are eaten (or drunk) by themselves.

So what is the role of sugar and sugary foods in the peak training diet? Using sugar well is a matter of choosing:

- the right amount (most of us could afford to cut our present intake by half, especially where kilojoules are in short supply);
- the right type (watch the fat–sugar combinations), and
- the right occasions (situations calling for a compact and low-fibre carbohydrate source).

While sugar and sugary foods generally fall into the category of 'less nutritious' carbohydrate sources, they often offer value in terms of being practical and enjoyable. Being compact, they can be added to a nutritious carbohydrate meal to boost the total carbohydrate content without adding extra bulk. At certain times, for example during an endurance event, the simplicity of a sports drink is all the nutrition that you need. And it is rare to find someone who doesn't like chocolate!

In the everyday training diet, when the big picture of your nutritional goals is important, sugar and less nutritious carbohydrate-rich foods should provide a small part of total energy intake. Even so, there may be occasions for specialised uses of these foods (e.g. a sports drink during and after prolonged training sessions). We shall see later that in many competition settings, overall nutritional goals can be overlooked in favour of practical and specialised uses of carbohydrate foods. In these situations, sugary foods may have a greater role to play in providing carbohydrate to the athlete.

## 1.4 Looking after your electrolytes

Salt is sodium chloride, with the the sodium portion of more interest to us here. Sodium is the most important electrolyte found outside the body's cells (potassium is its opposite partner within the cells). The sodium concentration helps to regulate blood pressure and volume, and assists in balancing the distribution of fluid and nutrients between the inside and outside of cells. When the sodium concentration falls outside its normal range, the delicate balance is disturbed and cell function can be crippled.

Your body has a fairly sophisticated system (involving amongst other things the kidneys and thirst drive) to regulate how much sodium and water is taken in, and how much these and the other electrolytes (potassium chloride, etc.) are excreted in urine. Electrolytes, particularly sodium, are also lost in other body fluids—the most important being sweat. Massive losses of sweat can potentially deplete the body's electrolyte stores, so the body cleverly adapts, with training and acclimatisation to a hot environment, by diluting your sweat and thus conserving electrolytes. It then expects you to replace nett losses through your diet. In this way, within a broad range of challenges the body can manage its electrolyte levels quite well.

However, the life of an athlete isn't always a series of gentle challenges, and it is probable that you throw your body into some extreme situations at times. Electrolyte balance can be threatened either by heavy consumption of electrolytes or by severe losses. The usual problem is overconsumption, and the usual culprit is sodium. In fact, the Australian diet has almost made excess salt intake an art form.

Sodium, like the other electrolytes, is found naturally in many foods. However, our dietary patterns have completely distorted sodium intake, through the addition of large amounts of salt to our foods and our meals. Other sodium compounds include MSG (monosodium glutamate), sodium bicarbonate, and some vitamin C tablets (sodium ascorbate). The kidneys battle hard with the excessive intake of sodium—however, one in five people will go on to suffer high blood pressure in later life. Excess salt also interferes with calcium balance and can contribute towards low bone density for those at risk. Since we don't always know who is at risk for these problems until it is too late, healthy nutrition guidelines encourage all Australians to curb their salt habits.

There is a much smaller possibility that salt depletion will occur, if massive sweat (and sodium) losses are not adequately replaced. Theoretically, this could happen if an unacclimatised athlete exercised furiously in a hot climate, with a restricted salt intake and plain water to replace fluid losses. In real life this happens rarely. A sports drink after long, sweaty sessions, or a little salt at the next meal will help to replace both fluid and electrolyte levels. It should be noted that today's sports drinks contain a relatively small amount of sodium, in the concentrations that can replace fluid and electrolytes simultaneously and in balance.

The need to replace sodium and electrolytes during exercise will be discussed in Chapter 4, which looks at competition. Your training sessions should follow a similar protocol, especially where they mimic the demands of strenuous competition.

One final word. Salt tablets are not necessary at any level or at any time. They provide more salt than the body can handle in one hit, and will provoke sodium–fluid imbalances, and frequently nausea and vomiting. Far from preventing or curing muscle cramps, they can be a disadvantage—even a danger—to your exercise per-formance.

### 1.5  *Replacing your daily fluid losses*

Water is your most important nutrient. The effects of dehydration are quickly felt and effect not only performance, but at times can endanger your life itself. The needs and strategies for fluid intake during exercise will be covered in Chapter 4: Competition. However, while athletes have become more aware of fluid needs in the competition arena, many completely forget about the training situation. It is an essential part of your training nutrition to look after day-to-day maintenance of fluid balance. Unfortunately, thirst is not a good indicator of what you need: you will have to work out what you are up against in your own training schedule, and plan your fluid strategies accordingly.

Depending on the length and intensity of training sessions, the acclimatisation of the athlete, and the environmental conditions, daily sweat losses can be considerable. In some cases, athletes will face greater dehydration threats in training than they will ever encounter

## HINTS FOR USING SALT WISELY

- Never take salt tablets.
- In general, there is no need to add salt to your food, either in cooking or at the table. Go easy also with salty sauces and flavourings (for example soy sauce, stock cubes and vegemite).
- Experiment with herbs, spices, lemon juice and other salt-free flavourings to make your meals tasty. Look at salt-free recipe books for ideas.
- Reduce your intake of salty snack foods, processed foods and take-aways.
- Learn to read labels to check the salt content of processed foods. Look for new varieties with reduced salt or low sodium content.
- Make this campaign a gradual process, and your taste buds will gradually adapt (and even thank you!).
- After lengthy training sessions in hot weather, you may be wise to drink a sports drink or add a little salt at your next meal—particularly until you adapt to the conditions.
- Practise your competition plans for fluid-electrolyte intake while in training—especially during prolonged intense sessions.

in competition. Swimmers, for instance, can train for hours in a warm pool and incur significant sweat losses, yet never become dehydrated in a 400 metre race!

It is especially tricky to comprehend dehydration in training when there is no visible proof of sweat. Swimmers are already wet, so how can they notice it? A cyclist might come home quite dry from a road session, because the sweat evaporates quickly in the passing wind.

One way to get an idea of your nett fluid loss is to weigh yourself before and after the session—each kilogram lost is roughly equal to a litre of fluid that must be replaced.

Another feature of training, unlike competition, is that conditions may not make fluid intake easy and accessible. There are no aid stations, and sometimes no trainers to bring out a water bottle to you. And if you are doing your long weekend run in the country, you are unlikely to come across a tap or a shop!

Looking after your fluid needs during training will mean better training (and greater improvement) as well as good practice for competition. You will be learning both to 'stomach' fluid while on the move, and to tolerate various sports drinks. And although the leading runners in the marathon make it look easy on television, there is quite a

21

---

HINTS FOR LOOKING AFTER FLUID NEEDS IN TRAINING

- Form a plan to look after your fluid needs. Don't leave it to good luck.

- Start a training session well-hydrated. On hot days, have an extra drink just before you start.

- Make fluids available during training sessions, especially during long sessions in hot weather.

- Include practice-runs for competition strategies—practise with the type, quantity and frequency of fluid intake that you intend to use during your event.

- Fully rehydrate between training sessions. Helpful strategies include keeping a jug of fluid in a prominent place that will remind you to drink.

- If you need a guide to your fluid deficit (and how much fluid should be replaced) after an exercise session, compare your pe- and post-body weight. (1kg loss is approximately equal to 1 litre of fluid.)

- Choose fluids that will help you meet other nutrition goals and be careful with the energy considerations. In most cases, water will be adequate.

- Monitoring morning bodyweight is a useful way to pick up chronic dehydration (often a sign of overtraining).

---

skill to grabbing a drink from an aid station and getting it all into your mouth without losing a stride.

You will also need to look at your fluid intake between training sessions to ensure that fluid levels have been fully restored. In most cases, water will be sufficient since your basic need is to replace fluid. However, fluids can also contain other nutrients, and depending on your individual situation, this can either be a useful way of supplying energy and other nutrients or a trap for overconsuming kilojoules.

Since liquids do not give you the same feeling of fullness as solid foods, it is usually easier to drink kilojoules than to eat them. This strategy can be useful for an athlete who needs help to meet massive daily energy needs, or who could benefit from carbohydrate intake straight after exercise but feels too tired or nauseous to eat. In other chapters you will see how drinks such as sports drinks, fruit juices and even soft drinks might become a carbohydrate vehicle, and 'liquid meals' can be made from low-fat milkshakes or special commercial supplements (such as Sustagen or Exceed Sports Nutrition Supplement). However, when your kilojoule needs are tight, you should concentrate on drinking water and low-energy fluid to replace fluid losses and save your kilojoules for food.

## 1.6  Using alcohol sensibly

Alcohol can be an enjoyable part of most lifestyles, including that of an athlete. It is hard to think of a celebration without champagne—and hopefully you will have many sports successes to celebrate! The issue with alcohol is how well you use it, and unfortunately in some sports alcohol is used very badly.

A nutrition text book will warn you about the health and social consequences of excessive alcohol intake, including its contribution to our annual road toll. For most athletes, however, tales of liver cirrhosis are hard to comprehend. But alcohol intake doesn't have to reach this level of abuse before it effects sports performance. With this in mind, we shall consider alcohol intake solely from the exercise viewpoint.

The immediate effects of drinking alcohol include dilation of blood vessels (vasodilation) and depression of the central nervous system. As a result, you will feel a little flushed (losing more heat through your skin) and your sensitivity will be dulled. So, while you think you are giving a great performance (be it in the disco or on the playing field), in actual fact your judgement, co-ordination and vision will be impaired. Effects will be related to the quantity of alcohol that you drink, and your individual tolerance (note that females tend to have poorer tolerance). However, most people will experience an effect after 20–30g of alcohol is consumed, and the effects will increase with the amount that is drunk. Figure 1.6 illustrates the alcohol content of various drinks.

Alcohol is not good for fluid replacement—in fact, it acts as a diuretic and may cause dehydration. And despite what you may have heard about beer and 'carbo-loading', alcoholic drinks will not fuel up your muscle glycogen stores. The kilojoules in alcoholic drinks come from alcohol, *not* carbohydrate, and alcohol is high in kilojoules—29 kJ per gram (see Figure 1.3). In addition, alcohol can interfere with glycogen synthesis.

The bottom line is that alcohol should not be consumed just prior to or during exercise (and this includes heavy intake on the night before sport). The penalties include dehydration, poor fuel stores, impaired skills, and a greater threat of hypothermia in a cold environment (heat losses though the skin will interfere with normal temperature regulation).

After exercise, alcohol intake should not compromise rehydration and refuelling needs. But, once these priorities are taken care of, there is only one other reason that could prevent athletes enjoying a couple of drinks. This issue, often forgotten in the post-match cheer, is the

**Figure 1.6 Alcohol content of common drinks**

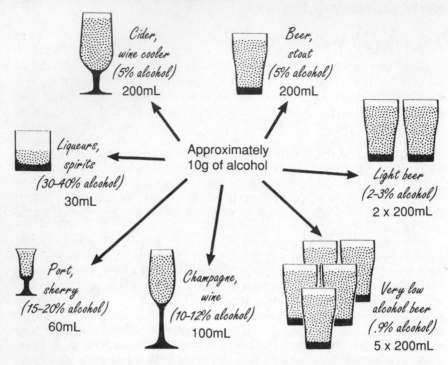

Cider,
wine cooler
(5% alcohol)
200mL

Beer,
stout
(5% alcohol)
200mL

Liqueurs,
spirits
(30–40% alcohol)
30mL

Approximately
10g of alcohol

Light beer
(2–3% alcohol)
2 x 200mL

Port,
sherry
(15–20% alcohol)
60mL

Champagne,
wine
(10–12% alcohol)
100mL

Very low
alcohol beer
(.9% alcohol)
5 x 200mL

vasodilatory effect of alcohol and its impact on tissue damage. Remember that you ice and elevate soft tissue injuries and bruising to constrict blood flow to the injured parts. The injured athlete who consumes alcohol immediately after the event may cause extra swelling and bleeding, delaying recovery, and in some cases even exacerbating the extent of the damage. The most sensible pathway for an injured athlete to take is to avoid any alcohol in the 24 hours post-exercise.

So should an athlete worry about occasional alcohol binges—or perhaps the weekly post-match 'wind-down'? The answer is that even a single episode of excess intake will cause some damage, and in particular will delay recovery and adaptation after exercise, and perhaps lengthen injury time. Slow recovery could be crucial if your next competition is a day, or even a week away, and catches you at less than your full capacity. Even if competition is sometime away, you should consider whether your next training sessions will be disrupted, and whether you can afford this.

The real problem with alcohol occurs when drinking binges are repeated, as is often seen in team sports after weekly matches. This

## HINTS FOR USING ALCOHOL SENSIBLY

- If you choose to drink alcohol, learn to enjoy a couple of glasses per occasion. It is much better to have a couple of drinks throughout the week, than save up for a binge on Saturday night (or after your competition).
- Avoid alcohol in the 24 hours prior to competition.
- Be wary of dehydration after consuming alcohol, as well as the increased risk of developing hypothermia in cold environments (e.g. skiing). Take precautions if you have consumed any alcohol prior to training sessions (including the night before).
- Enjoy alcohol after competition, without causing damage to yourself or your performance. Rehydrate and refuel with carbohydrates before you start with alcoholic drinks, then set yourself a limit and be aware of how much you have consumed. Don't get caught up in group drinking situations. The advice which accompanies drink-driving laws in your state may be a useful guide (see Figure 1.6 for a guide to the alcohol content of drinks).
- Avoid any alcohol for 24 hours post-exercise if any soft tissue injuries or bruising have occurred.
- Use tricks to make the alcohol go further. Drink low-alcohol beers, mix your wine with mineral water and order half-nips of spirits in mixed drinks. Make plenty of non-alcoholic drinks available, both as thirst-quenchers and as an enjoyable alternative to alcohol. This could include fruit juices, plain mineral water, and soft drinks, as well as special non-alcoholic cocktails.
- If you need to restrict your energy intake, treat alcohol as a luxury item. There are more nutritious ways of consuming kilojoules.

will slowly but surely erode your skills, your fitness and your sports career. And that is a fact—even if everyone on the team does it and it appears to be normal (or desirable) behaviour. Another thing to remember is that alcohol is a high-kilojoule source of poor nutritional value. Heavy consumption and binge periods will lead to weight gain. Have you noticed how much heavier you are on your return from the end-of-season trip?

Alcohol is not 'sweated out' or 'exercised off'—these are just more of the locker room tales that help to sustain alcohol misuse in sports. It is a drug that at high levels causes damage to many organs and tissues in your body. The only way to prevent this from happening is not to drink to excess.

Having said all this, alcohol can be a small part of a healthy diet. A drink after a hard day's training can help you relax, and a few drinks can add sparkle to social occasions. If you choose to drink, make it work for you, rather than pull your sports potential back to the level of those who would have you believe that 'team bonding' (getting drunk together) is all that sport has to offer.

# 2 Fine tuning—how much and when?

Now that the basic principles are in place, it is time to start accounting for your individual characteristics, and to plan for your specific needs. You must calculate your requirements for the various nutrients, and then arrange these within your energy budget. And of course, you will need to consider how best to arrange your food intake over your busy day—to gain nutritional advantages as well as meet your schedule of commitments.

## 2.1 Energy

How many kilojoules should I eat each day? This is a question frequently thrown at dietitians—and athletes expect an answer to three decimal places. Such precision is impossible, because your body is a unique energy system with its own tally of energy needs. In a nutshell, you need enough energy to be you!

The major factors that make up your total energy requirements are:

- Your resting metabolic rate—the energy required just to keep your body functioning. This varies with age (decreasing as you get older), with body mass (increasing with a larger body mass), with body composition (increasing with greater muscle mass and decreasing with greater fat stores), and gender (greater in men than women). Metabolic rate is determined and altered by many other factors as well.

  Obviously, this energy need will vary greatly between people, and can be a great source of frustration and discouragement to those who 'drew the short end of the stick'. We all know those lucky people who can eat food by the truckload without gaining a gram of body fat (due to an inefficient metabolism which 'wastes' food energy), while others horde every kilojoule they are presented with (efficient metabolism) and gain a kilo just by smelling a box of chocolates!

- Growth, including pregnancy and breast-feeding. Children and adolescents may need plenty of additional kilojoules to provide for new bone and body tissues as they grow.

27

**Figure 2.1 How to predict your daily energy requirements**

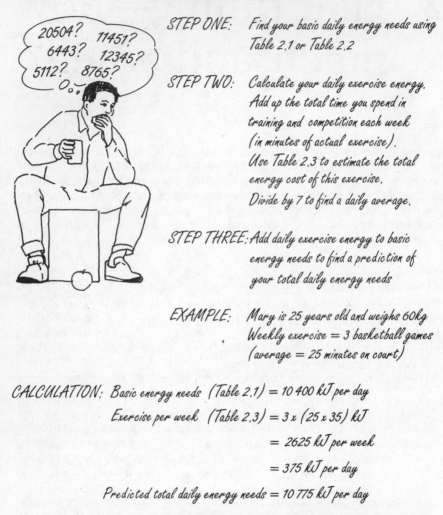

STEP ONE: *Find your basic daily energy needs using Table 2.1 or Table 2.2*

STEP TWO: *Calculate your daily exercise energy. Add up the total time you spend in training and competition each week (in minutes of actual exercise). Use Table 2.3 to estimate the total energy cost of this exercise. Divide by 7 to find a daily average.*

STEP THREE: *Add daily exercise energy to basic energy needs to find a prediction of your total daily energy needs*

EXAMPLE: *Mary is 25 years old and weighs 60kg Weekly exercise = 3 basketball games (average = 25 minutes on court)*

CALCULATION: *Basic energy needs (Table 2.1) = 10 400 kJ per day*

*Exercise per week (Table 2.3) = 3 x (25 x 35) kJ*

*= 2625 kJ per week*

*= 375 kJ per day*

*Predicted total daily energy needs = 10 775 kJ per day*

- Muscular work. While some athletes hold jobs that involve heavy manual labour, for the most part it is exercise, and particularly the training schedule, that adds a significant contribution to total energy needs.

So how can you tell what your total energy requirements will be? An approximation can be made using tables that calculate average figures for each of these major factors. Remember, however, that individuals vary quite remarkably around average figures, and that the purpose of doing such a calculation will be to find a ballpark figure for your expected energy requirements. See Figure 2.1 for instructions on how to calculate your estimated energy needs. Don't be surprised or disappointed if your estimation doesn't seem to match exactly your usual energy intake from food. (After all, you probably don't earn the average wage in this country either).

Most of the time, we want to be in energy balance (this is when we match our energy requirements with a similar intake of energy from food). Your body has a buffer for this energy balance equation. The body's fat stores provide an energy reserve to store extra kilojoules when you consume more than you expend, or to make up the deficit when the reverse is true. This is how you gain or lose weight from body fat. (See Figure 2.2)

Even when you are in energy balance (neither gaining or losing body fat), you will not necessarily have to eat *exactly* the same number of kilojoules as you expend for that day. In the short term—say over a couple of days—there may be little correlation between your energy input and requirements. However over a period of a week or more, the energy balance equation should be maintained with considerable precision.

This gives you a way of fine-tuning the assessment of your energy requirements. If you can record your total food intake for a week, accurately and honestly, without changing things just because you are watching yourself, then an assessment of your energy intake will give you a closer estimation of your energy requirements (energy intake equals energy requirement, right?) Remember, you must be following your usual habits, and neither gain nor lose body fat over this time. A dietitian can instruct you how to undertake this task, and will make an expert analysis of the results. (The dietary analysis can also tell you about your intake of carbohydrate, protein, vitamins and minerals, making it a valuable exercise.)

Your energy requirements are individual and specific to you. In general, the greatest (estimated) energy requirements belong to athletes who are young, growing, large, with plenty of muscle mass, and who undertake lengthy intense training sessions each day. Into this category we might put giant teenage basketballers, heavyweight rowers, marathon runners and triathletes. On the other hand females will be expected to have smaller energy requirements, and a tiny athlete who does little training (or training that is skill-based rather than energy-intensive) will be the typical small-energy consumer. Female gymnasts and ballet dancers are a good example.

These generalisations are by no means hard and fast. You should not be surprised if your predicted (tables) and estimated (food diary) energy requirements are quite different from other athletes—even those in the same sport as you. The most important thing is that they are right for you.

**Figure 2.2 Energy balance**

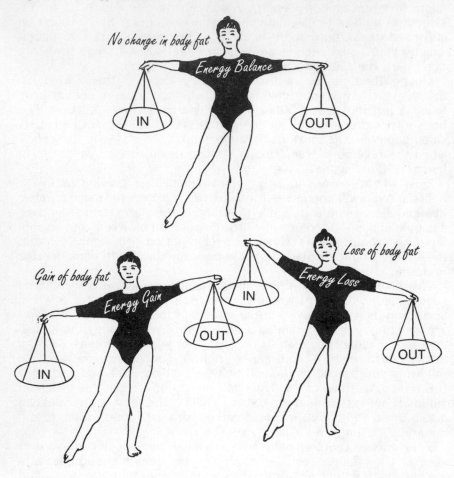

Once you have an idea of your daily kilojoule budget, your next task is to see how you can 'spend' it wisely to ensure that you cover your requirements for the following important nutrients.

## 2.2 Carbohydrate

Your carbohydrate requirements are estimated on the basis of muscle glycogen needs, to replace the fuel that you burn up in daily exercise. This will depend on the amount of training (or competition) that you undertake each day, and the size of your muscles.

**Table 2.1  Estimated daily energy allowances for reference adults**

|  | Your body weight | Daily energy (kilojoules/day[a]) | | |
|---|---|---|---|---|
|  |  | 25 yrs | 45 yrs | 65 yrs |
| Men | 55kg | 9 800 | 9 200 | 7 600 |
|  | 60kg | 10 400 | 9 600 | 8 000 |
|  | 65kg | 11 000 | 10 000 | 8 400 |
|  | 70kg | 11 600 | 10 400 | 8 800 |
|  | 75kg | 12 200 | 10 800 | 9 200 |
|  | 80kg | 12 800 | 11 200 | 9 600 |
|  | 85kg | 13 400 | 11 600 | 10 000 |
|  | 90kg | 14 600 | 12 400 | 10 800 |
| Women | 40kg | 7 000 | 6 200 | 5 800 |
|  | 45kg | 7 400 | 6 600 | 6 000 |
|  | 50kg | 7 800 | 7 000 | 6 200 |
|  | 55kg | 8 200 | 7 400 | 6 400 |
|  | 60kg | 8 600 | 7 800 | 6 600 |
|  | 65kg | 9 000 | 8 200 | 6 800 |
|  | 70kg | 9 400 | 8 600 | 7 000 |
|  | 75kg | 9 800 | 9 000 | 7 200 |

**Table 2.2  Estimated daily energy allowances for growth. Pregnancy and breastfeeding**

|  |  | Daily energy (kilojoules/day[a]) | |
|---|---|---|---|
| Boys | 11–15 yrs | (41kg) | 12 200 |
|  | 15–18 yrs | (61kg) | 12 600 |
| Girls | 11–15 yrs | (42kg) | 10 400 |
|  | 15–18 yrs | (55kg) | 9 200 |
| Pregnancy | Trimesters 2 & 3 |  | 8 200 |
| Breastfeeding | 18–35 yrs |  | 10 900 |
|  | 35+ |  | 10 100 |

*Note*:  [a] Kilocalories can be calculated by dividing by 4.2
*Source*:  *Dietary allowances for use in Australia*. AGPS: Canberra, 1987

A general estimation of the daily carbohydrate needs of various athletes is as follows:

General sports activity (up to 60 minutes of training per day or unlimited low-intensity training)   5–6g of carbohydrate for each kg you weigh

Moderately training athletes (60–120 minutes of intense or lengthy medium-intensity exercise)   6–8g of carbohydrate for each kg you weigh

Endurance training (Over 120 minutes of intense training per day)   9–10g+ of carbohydrate for each kg you weigh

| Extreme exercise—(5–6+ hours of intense daily exercise—e.g. cycle tour) | 12–13g of carbohydrate for each kg you weigh |

So a female basketballer (60kg) whose daily training added up to 30–60 minutes of actual exercise would have approximate carbohydrate needs of 300–360g per day. A 65kg triathlete training strenuously for 3–4 hours each day should aim for 585–650g of carbohydrate each day to replace carbohydrate stores. Look at Table 2.4 for a ready-reckoner of carbohydrate content of various foods. According to this guide, our triathlete would need to eat around 40 'serves' of carbohydrate foods each day—for example 2 large bowls of cereal (8 serves), 12 slices of bread (12), 8 pieces of fruit (8), 3 cups of juice (6) and 3 cups of cooked pasta (6)!

Clearly, carbohydrate will take up most of the kilojoules in your diet. In fact, it is estimated that carbohydrate may account for the following percentages of total energy intake:

| General and moderate training level | 50–60 per cent of total energy |
| Endurance training | 60–70 per cent of total energy |
| Restricted energy diet (low energy consumers and weight loss diets) | 60–70 per cent of total energy |

While these figures are only a general guide, they reflect how far you may need to change your dietary patterns from a typical Australian diet (currently providing 40–45 per cent of energy as carbohydrate).

Do you need to count up your carbohydrate intake each day? For most athletes this is probably an unnecessary task. The food hints summarised in Chapter 1.3 should help you form habits that will increase your carbohydrate intake to the 50–60 per cent energy mark. Athletes who have to push their carbohydrate and total kilojoule intakes further may be helped by periodically calculating the amount of carbohydrate foods needed, because it is often more than their appetites or typical meal patterns would 'naturally' achieve. In a special situation such as carbo-loading, when you need to maximise glycogen storage, carbohydrate counting will ensure that you achieve your daily target of 9–10g per kilogram of your weight.

### 2.3 Protein

The protein needs of athletes have been hotly debated for many years. In the red corner, we have strength sports who argue that large intakes of protein are needed for great big muscles! And in the black corner, we have endurance athletes who get so involved in

**Table 2.3  Estimated energy cost of activity (kilojoules/minute)**

| Activity | | Your body weight | | | | |
|---|---|---|---|---|---|---|
| | | 50kg | 60kg | 70kg | 80kg | 90kg |
| Aerobics | *beginners* | 22 | 26 | 30 | 34 | 39 |
| | *advanced* | 28 | 33 | 40 | 45 | 51 |
| Badminton | | 20 | 24 | 28 | 33 | 37 |
| Ballroom dancing | | 11 | 13 | 15 | 17 | 19 |
| Basketball | | 29 | 35 | 40 | 46 | 52 |
| Boxing | *sparring* | 46 | 56 | 65 | 74 | 84 |
| | *in ring* | 29 | 35 | 40 | 46 | 52 |
| Canoeing | *leisure* | 9 | 11 | 13 | 15 | 17 |
| | *racing* | 22 | 26 | 30 | 34 | 39 |
| Circuit training | | 22 | 26 | 30 | 34 | 40 |
| Cricket | *batting* | 17 | 21 | 24 | 28 | 32 |
| | *bowling* | 19 | 22 | 26 | 30 | 34 |
| Cycling | *9 km/hr* | 13 | 16 | 18 | 21 | 24 |
| | *15 km/hr* | 21 | 24 | 28 | 33 | 38 |
| | *racing* | 35 | 42 | 49 | 56 | 63 |
| Football | | 28 | 33 | 39 | 44 | 50 |
| Golf | | 18 | 21 | 25 | 28 | 32 |
| Gymnastics | | 14 | 16 | 19 | 22 | 25 |
| Hockey | | 18 | 20 | 24 | 29 | 33 |
| Judo | | 41 | 49 | 57 | 65 | 73 |
| Running | *5.5 min per km* | 40 | 49 | 57 | 65 | 73 |
| | *5 min per km* | 44 | 52 | 61 | 70 | 78 |
| | *4.5 min per km* | 48 | 55 | 65 | 75 | 85 |
| | *4 min per km* | 54 | 65 | 76 | 87 | 98 |
| Skiing | *cross-country* | 35 | 42 | 49 | 56 | 63 |
| | *down hill (easy)* | 18 | 21 | 25 | 29 | 33 |
| | *down hill (hard)* | 29 | 35 | 40 | 49 | 55 |
| Squash | | 44 | 53 | 62 | 71 | 79 |
| Swimming | *freestyle* | 33 | 40 | 46 | 52 | 59 |
| | *backstroke* | 36 | 43 | 49 | 56 | 63 |
| | *breastroke* | 34 | 41 | 47 | 54 | 61 |
| Table tennis | | 14 | 17 | 19 | 23 | 26 |
| Tennis | *social* | 15 | 17 | 20 | 23 | 26 |
| | *competitive* | 37 | 44 | 50 | 58 | 65 |
| Volleyball | | 10 | 12 | 15 | 17 | 19 |
| Walking | *10 min per km* | 21 | 26 | 30 | 35 | 39 |
| | *8 min per km* | 25 | 30 | 35 | 40 | 45 |
| | *5 min per km* | 44 | 52 | 61 | 70 | 78 |
| **Adjustment for occupational activity**—adjust total daily energy allowance | | | | | | |
| Minimum daily activity (e.g. bedridden, wheelchair) | | −2000 | −2400 | −2800 | −3200 | −3600 |
| Heavy labouring job | | +2000 | +2400 | +2800 | +3200 | +3600 |

*Notes:*  All figures are approximate values only.
   Kilocalories can be calculated by dividing kilojoule values by 4.2
*Source:*  Adapted from: *Recommended nutrient intakes*, NHMRC: Australia, 1990
   Katch F.I. and McArdle W.D., *Nutrition, Weight Control and Exercise*, Lea and Febiger: Philadelphia 1988

**Table 2.4   Ready reckoner of carbohydrate-rich foods**

Approximately 15g of carbohydrate is supplied by the following foods:

| | | |
|---|---|---|
| Cereals | bread | 1 thick slice (40g) |
| | bread roll | 1/2 average roll (35g) |
| | muffin or crumpet | 1/2 average (35g) |
| | breakfast cereal | 20g = 1/2 to 2/3 cup Weeties or 'light' cereal |
| | | = 1/3 cup muesli flakes or 'heavier' cereal |
| | | = 1.5 Weetbix |
| | rolled oats | 1/4 cup (20g) |
| | untoasted muesli | 1/4 cup (20g) |
| | porridge | 3/4 cup cooked (180g) |
| | scones/pancakes | 30g = 1/2 average size |
| | wholemeal cake (low fat) | 25g = 1/2 to 1/3 av. slice |
| | dry biscuit | 25g = 4–6 crackers |
| | rice cakes | 15g = 1.5 cakes |
| | plain muesli bar | 20g = 2/3 bar |
| | plain sweet biscuit | 20g = 2 |
| | popcorn | 20g = 1 cup |
| | rice | 1/3 cup cooked (50g) |
| | pasta/noodles | 1/2 cup cooked (60g) |
| Vegetables | potatoes | 80g cooked (1 med) |
| | | 90g mashed (1/3 cup) |
| | carrots/pumpkin/peas | 300g cooked (1.5 cups) |
| | corn | 70g cooked (1/2 cup) |
| Legumes | kidney, soy beans | 1/3 cup cooked (80g) |
| | baked beans | 3/5 cup (150g) |
| | lentils | 1/3 cup cooked (80g) |
| Fruit | fresh fruit | 100–150g piece |
| | | = medium apple, orange |
| | | = small banana |
| | | = 3/4 cup cherries, grapes |
| | juice | 120ml sweetened (1/2 cup) |
| | | 180ml unsweetened (3/4 cup) |
| | dried fruit | 20g (1.5 Tablespoons) |
| | canned/stewed fruit | 120g sweetened (1/2 cup) |
| | | 240g unsweetened (1 cup) |
| | fruit salad, fresh | 120g (1/2 cup) |
| Dairy products | skim milk | 300ml |
| | fruit non-fat yoghurt | 100g (1/2 carton) |
| | plain non-fat yoghurt | 200g (carton) |
| | low-fat icecream | 100g (2 rounded Tablespoons) |
| Sugary foods | sugar | 15g (2 heaped teaspoons) |
| | jam and honey | 20g (Tablespoon) |
| | plain lollies | 15–20g packet |
| Drinks | soft drinks and flavoured min. water | 150ml |
| | cordial | 200ml |
| | fruit juice | 120–180ml |
| | sports drinks | 200–250ml |
| | liquid meal drinks | 100ml |
| | carbo-loader drinks | 100ml |
| | low-fat milk shakes | 120–150ml |

*Source*:   NUTTAB 1990, Australian Department of Community Services and Health carbohydrate counting that they shun protein altogether. Luckily, in recent years sufficient scientific research has allowed the referee to step into the ring with a final verdict.

And the decision is: protein requirements *are* increased by exercise—firstly to account for the small contribution of protein to muscle fuel, and secondly to account for any extra muscle that is laid down. However, don't go rushing for a protein powder—although protein requirements increase in absolute terms (you may need more total grams), the extra kilojoules in your diet will automatically allow you to eat more protein without having to consciously emphasise protein foods.

In fact, for many athletes, total protein needs will still be met by the general recommendation of 1g of protein per kilogram of body weight—e.g. 60g for a 60kg athlete. But athletes whose daily training sessions are lengthy and intense (burning up a significant total of protein fuel), or who are in a muscle gain stage of their programs, will require an increase in their protein allowance. Athletes who are growing will need to cover these physiological requirements as well. The protein requirements for various groups of athletes might be summarised as follows:

| | |
|---|---|
| General sports activity | 1g of protein for every kg you weigh |
| Strength-training athletes (aim for the high end of range during muscle gain periods) | 1.2–1.5g of protein for every kg you weigh |
| Endurance training athletes (aim for the high end of range for very prolonged strenuous training) | 1.2–1.6g of protein for every kg you weigh |
| Adolescent and growing athletes | 2.0g of protein for every kg you weigh |
| Pregnant athletes | Extra 10g of protein per day in trimesters 2 and 3 |
| Breast-feeding athletes | Extra 20g of protein per day |

In general, you should earmark about 12–15 per cent of your total energy intake to meet these recommended levels—the same as most Australians do now. Even at this level, most athletes who eat a high-energy intake will surpass these daily protein amounts. However low-energy consumers may find that 15–20 per cent of their total energy budget is needed.

Protein foods should be chosen with your other nutritional goals in mind—that is, you should choose protein foods with a minimal fat

**Table 2.5   Ready reckoner of protein-rich foods**

Approximately 10g of protein is provided by the following foods:

| Low-fat animal foods | grilled fish | 50g (cooked weight) |
|---|---|---|
| | tuna or salmon | 50g |
| | lean beef or lamb | 35g (cooked weight) |
| | veal | 35g (cooked weight) |
| | turkey or chicken | 40g (cooked weight) |
| | game meat (rabbit, venison) | 35g (cooked weight) |
| | eggs | 2 small |
| | cottage cheese | 70g |
| | reduced-fat cheese (11% fat slices) | 30g = 1.5sl |
| | non-fat fruit yoghurt | 200g carton |
| | skim milk | 300ml |
| | liquid meal supplement (Sustagen or Exceed Sports Nutrition Supplement) | 150ml |
| Vegetable foods | wholemeal bread | 4sl (120g) |
| | wheat flake cereal | 3 cups (90g) |
| | untoasted muesli | 1 cup (100g) |
| | cooked pasta or noodles | 2 cups (300g) |
| | cooked brown rice | 3 cups (400g) |
| | cooked lentils | 3/4 cup (150g) |
| | cooked kidney beans | 3/4 cup (150g) |
| | baked beans | 4/5 cup (200g) |
| | cooked soy beans or tofu | 120g |
| | nuts | 60g |
| | seeds (e.g. sesame) | 60g |

*Source*:   NUTTAB 1990, Australian Department of Community Services and Health

content which are also good sources of other nutrients. Table 2.5 provides a ready reckoner of the protein content of some valuable foods. Lean animal protein foods are able to supply all the body's essential amino acids, as well as calcium (dairy foods) and iron (meats and shellfish). If you look at the vegetable protein foods, you will see that some of these appear as good carbohydrate sources also. The ready reckoner should convince you that it doesn't take half a side of beef to make up your daily protein needs—cereal with skim milk for breakfast, a chicken sandwich for lunch and a small steak for dinner will provide over 60g of protein for a 60kg squash player.

Is vegetable protein as valuable as animal protein? Protein is made from various combinations of small building blocks called amino acids. Some of these amino acids can be manufactured in the body by rearranging the structure of other compounds, while the other amino acids (called the essential amino acids) can only be obtained by eating food. Animal protein foods contain a good variety of amino acids including all the essentials ones. On the other hand, plant foods tend to have one or more of the essential amino acids in short supply. This could be a problem if plant foods make up most or all of your diet— for example if you are a vegetarian.

Fortunately however, while one vegetable protein food will contain

**Figure 2.3 By combining certain food groups, vegetable protein foods are complemented and a first-class protein meal is achieved**

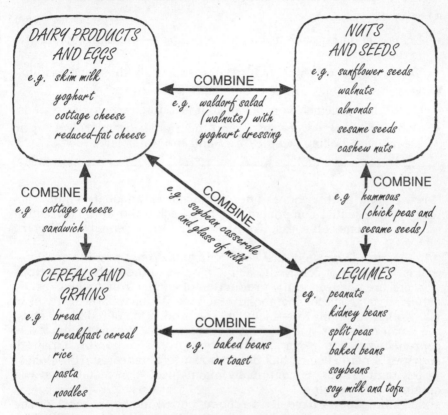

a good supply of some essential amino acids, while lacking in one or two others, another vegetable protein food will have the reverse problem. By cleverly mixing and matching these foods the total amino acid picture can be achieved. This is known as *complementing* vegetable proteins, and can also be done by mixing a vegetable type with a small amount of animal protein, such as a dairy food. Figure 2.3 shows you which protein foods can complement each other, and some typical examples.

### 2.4 Vitamins

Helped along by some clever advertising from vitamin supplement companies, most people think of vitamins as the most important nutrients in their diet and the ones most likely to run into short supply.

---

## HINTS FOR PUTTING MORE VITAMINS PER MOUTHFUL IN YOUR DIET

- Enjoy a good range of fruits and vegetables—the more colour the better.
- Where possible choose fresh types, especially those in season.
- Frozen vegetables are also a nutritious choice.
- Go for the wholemeal versions of your favourite carbohydrate foods.
- Don't overcook vegetables—keep them crisp by microwaving or steaming. If boiling, keep it brief and the water level low.

---

However, the truth is quite different. While an adequate vitamin intake is an essential component of good health and optimal training nutrition it is one of the least likely things to be deficient in the Western diet.

In the correct sense of the word, vitamins do not provide energy—that is, they do not contribute any kilojoules to the body. But various vitamins are involved in the production of energy from fuel stores, by acting as catalysts for metabolic reactions. Vitamins are involved in many other reactions too—including the production of red blood cells, the repair of tissues, and the synthesis of protein. When vitamin levels drop below a certain mark, these body processes will be impaired, and sports performance has been shown to be affected. However, if your vitamin supply is continually maintained, then metabolism will continue unimpeded.

Nutrition experts have set a recommended intake for most of the vitamins (known as the Recommended Dietary Intake or RDI). The RDIs for vitamins are set as a general target, and most peoples' diets provide intakes well above these levels. A diet that provides less than the RDI for a vitamin is not necessarily deficient in that vitamin, because quite a large safety margin has been set.

However, if your usual diet consistently supplies you with less than two-thirds of the RDIs, some expert dietary advice and remodelling is suggested. The first line of attack will *not* be to take a vitamin supplement, but rather to change your diet to overcome its shortfalls. After all, because nutrients exist together in food, it is likely that any diet that is low in one or more vitamins also fails to meet other goals of peak training nutrition. A vitamin supplement might reverse your low vitamin intake, but how will it help your high fat intake or your low carbohydrate supply?

After looking at the population RDIs for vitamins, athletes usually ask two questions:

- Does heavy exercise increase the requirements for vitamins?
- Will extra vitamins, especially large doses, improve performance by making metabolism move faster?

The second question really belongs in the area of supplements and ergogenic aids (performance boosters), and will be covered in Chapter 6. On the trail of extra vitamin needs, research has not been able to show that the vitamin requirements of athletes are raised above the RDI levels. In fact, the RDIs for the vitamins involved in energy metabolism have been set according to energy intake level. So a higher energy expenditure already has an inbuilt increase in total vitamin requirement.

Table 2.6 summarises food sources of each vitamin, with RDIs adjusted for athletes. Where an RDI has not been set for a vitamin, it is assumed that an adequate intake is already taken care of. In terms of vitamin intake, the two biggest assets that an athlete's diet can have are a high energy intake (more food should mean more nutrients), and a wide variety of foods (as you learnt earlier, variety increases your opportunities to get a little of everything you need).

Athletes most likely to run into problems with vitamin intake are those on very restricted diets (e.g. fad diets, strict vegetarian diets, fussy eaters) and those with low energy intakes (low energy consumers and weight loss diets). In these situations, a sports dietitian can help you to maximise your dietary intake, and may also suggest a low-dose vitamin supplement to help fill any remaining gaps.

## 2.5 Iron

Iron is an important nutrient in sports performance, since it is a component of the oxygen carriers in the blood (called hemoglobin) and in the muscles (called myoglobin). In addition, iron is involved with some of the enzymes that promote exercise metabolism. An iron deficiency will reduce the oxygen supply to muscles as well as slow down some of these metabolic reactions. Obviously, this is not compatible with optimal performance.

Athletes with very low iron stores complain of tiredness and poor recovery from training. If the situation worsens and blood hemoglobin levels become lowered (called anemia) the symptoms become more drastic—severe fatigue, cramps, headaches and often shortness of breath. It is at the anemia stage that there is definite proof of reduced performance. Even if low iron stores do not directly cause changes to performance, they are generally treated to stop the progression to anemia.

Iron requirements for athletes provide a few challenges. Firstly, females need to eat more iron than their male counterparts to counter the blood losses of menstruation. The tricky part is that females

**Table 2.6 Vitamins: where to find your recommended dietary intake (RDI)**

| Vitamins | Daily RDI for adult athletes | Good dietary sources | Examples of RDI from food |
|---|---|---|---|
| Thiamin (vitamin B1) | 0.10mg per 1000 kJ that you eat<br>i.e. 6 000 kJ = 0.6mg<br>10 000 kJ = 1.0mg<br>20 000 kJ = 2.0mg | Pork, liver (& pate) breakfast cereals, wholegrain breads and cereal foods, yeast extract, legumes (e.g. Vegemite) | 1mg is provided by:<br>2 slices wholemeal bread<br>+ 1 tsp Vegemite<br>+ 1 cup Weeties |
| Riboflavin (vitamin B2) | 0.15mg per 1000 kJ that you eat<br>i.e. 6 000 kJ = 0.9mg<br>10 000 kJ = 1.5mg<br>20 000 kJ = 3.0mg | Liver, dairy products, breakfast cereals, yeast extract, wholemeal breads and cereal foods | 1.5mg is provided by:<br>2 Weetbix<br>+ 1 cup skim milk<br>+ 2 slices wholemeal bread<br>+ 200g carton low-fat yoghurt |
| Niacin (vitamin B3) | 1.6mg per 1000 kJ that you eat<br>i.e. 6 000 kJ = 9.6mg<br>10 000 kJ = 16mg<br>20 000 kJ = 32mg | Meats/eggs/fish/dairy foods, yeast extract, breakfast cereals, wholegrain breads and cereal foods legumes | 16mg is provided by:<br>2 slices wholemeal bread<br>+ 120g lean meat<br>+ 1 cup skim milk |
| Pyridoxine (vitamin B6) | 0.02mg per gram of protein that you eat<br>i.e. 50g protein = 1.0mg<br>100g protein = 2.0mg | High protein foods, wholegrain breads and cereal foods, potatoes, bananas | 1mg is provided by:<br>1 banana<br>+ 1 cup Allbran<br>+ 100g chicken |
| Folate | 200µg | Green leafy vegies, oranges, wholegrain breads + cereal foods, liver | 200µg is provided by:<br>200ml orange juice + 1 cup spinach |
| Pantothenic acid | No RDI—widely distributed | Meats/fish/egg, wholegrain breads + cereal foods, legumes | Widely distributed in foods |

| | | | |
|---|---|---|---|
| Biotin | No RDI—some manufactured by gut bacteria | Liver, meats, egg yolks, nuts | — |
| Vitamin B12 | 2mcg | Animal foods—not generally found in plant foods. | Small amount of animal foods |
| Ascorbic acid (vitamin C) | 30mg (women) 40mg (men) | Citrus fruits, berries, tropical fruits, tomato, green leafy vegetables, parsley | 40mg is provided by: half an orange or 1/2 cup fresh strawberries |
| Vitamin A | 750µg | Liver (& pate), dairy products, some fish, green leafy vegetables, yellow/ orange fruits and vegetables (carrots, peaches, spinach etc). | 750µg is provided by: 1/2 cup cooked carrots or 1 mango |
| Vitamin D | Manufactured by the action of sunlight on skin | Butter/margarine, fish oils, eggs | Daily sunlight |
| Vitamin E | 10mg | Wheatgerm and wholegrain cereal foods, nuts, seeds, vegetable oils, margarine, avocado | 10mg is provided by: 1 avocado + Tbs peanut butter + 2 tsp polyunsaturated margarine + cup untoasted muesli |
| Vitamin K | No RDI—some manufactured by gut bacteria | Liver, green leafy vegetables: cabbage, cauliflower, broccoli, legumes | — |

Source: Recommended nutrient intakes, Australia NHMRC, 1990

usually need to eat less kilojoules than males, and must therefore find more iron per mouthful in their diet.

Secondly, heavy exercise increases iron requirements, by increasing iron losses from the body. Iron can be lost through sweat and gastrointestinal bleeding—particularly if you take a lot of anti-inflammatory drugs for injuries. Red blood cells are destroyed by continual jarring and impact, whether in contact sports or from pounding the pavements while running. A guide to iron requirements is provided as follows. The upper ranges for the endurance athletes represent the worst-case scenario where an athlete is experiencing iron loss from all exercise issues:

General training—males and non-menstruating females — 7mg iron per day

General training—menstruating females — 12–16mg iron per day

General training—growing adolescents — 10–13mg iron per day

Pregnancy (trimesters 2 and 3) — 22–36mg iron per day

Endurance training—males (particularly running and other high-impact sports) — 7–17.5mg iron per day

Endurance training—non-menstruating females (particularly high-impact sports) — 7–17mg iron per day

Endurance training—menstruating females (particularly high-impact sports) — 16–23mg iron per day

**Table 2.7  Iron-rich foods for the optimal training diet**

| Food | Serve | mg Iron |
|---|---|---|
| ✳Heme iron foods | | |
| liver | 100g (cooked weight) | 11.0mg |
| liver pate | 40g (2 Tbsp) | 2–3mg |
| lean steak | 100g (cooked weight) | 4.0mg |
| chicken (dark meat) | 100g (cooked weight) | 1.2mg |
| fish | 100g (cooked weight) | 0.6–1.4mg |
| oysters | 100g | 3.9mg |
| salmon | 100g (small tin) | 1.5mg |
| Non-heme iron foods | | |
| eggs | 100g (2) | 2.0mg |
| breakfast cereal (fortified) | 30g (1 cup) | 2.5mg |
| wholemeal bread | 60g (2 sl) | 1.4mg |
| spinach (cooked) | 145g (1 cup) | 4.4mg |
| lentils/kidney beans (cooked) | 100g (2/3 cup) | 2.5mg |
| tofu | 100g | 1.9mg |
| sultanas | 50g | 0.9mg |
| dried apricots | 50g | 2.0mg |
| almonds | 50g | 2.1mg |

*Source*: NUTTAB 1990, Australian Department of Community Services and Health

---

## HINTS FOR AN IRON BOOST

- Include lean red meat or liver (pate, perhaps) in your meals three to five times per week. It doesn't have to be a big serve—perhaps a slice in a sandwich or a handful in your stir-fry. These foods not only contribute heme iron (well-absorbed), but they increase the absorption of non-heme iron from other foods at the same meal.

- Other sources of heme iron are seafood (especially oysters) darker types of fish, and the dark cuts of poultry (the leg rather than the breast). Like meat, they can be used to enhance the total iron absorbed from the meal.

- Make use of commercial breakfast cereals that have been fortified with iron.

- If you are not having a heme iron food at a meal, make sure that you have a good serve of a non-heme iron food—such as eggs, a wholegrain cereal food, some legumes or some spinach/silverbeet.

  *AND*

  Combine these non-heme iron meals with a vitamin C food to enhance the iron absorption—for example, orange juice with your breakfast cereal, tomatoes with your spinach omelette.

- Avoid sprinkling wheat bran on your meals. You probably don't need extra fibre in your peak training diet.

- Don't drink strong tea with your meals if you are in a high risk category for iron deficiency.

- Work extra hard on the non-heme mixes and matches if you are a vegetarian, and think about cooking in cast iron pots.

---

The final complication in the iron situation is that the people who need to eat the highest intakes are often the people who steer away from the most valuable foods. Dietary iron is found in two forms—a special form called 'heme' iron that occurrs in some animal foods, and a simpler form known as 'non-heme' iron. Table 2.7 shows the iron content of some common serves of food.

The importance of this classification is two-fold—the heme foods have generally more iron overall and, secondly, the heme iron is well absorbed. By contrast, the non-heme iron is poorly absorbed, and can be further tied up by other factors in food such as tannin (in tea), phytates (in wheat bran and wholemeal cereals) and oxalates (in spinach). Athletes whose diets are based heavily, or solely, on plant iron foods—such as vegetarians or endurance athletes who are keen on carbohydrates only—may find that their iron intake is inadequate and unavailable.

Some special tactics are needed to put an iron boost into the optimal training diet. This will include clever mixing and matching of foods to make use of low-fat heme iron foods, and to take advantage of dietary factors that actually enhance the absorption of non-heme iron—vitamin C and meat/fish/poultry itself.

### 2.6 Calcium

The best-known function of calcium in the body is its role in the making up bone, since 99 per cent of the body's calcium is in the skeleton.

A growing awareness of osteoporosis has put the spotlight on calcium in recent years. Osteoporosis is typically a process of ageing, more pronounced in women, which leaves bones thinner and more fragile. Remember how your grandmother fell and broke her hip or her arm? The most influential factor in loss of bone calcium is thought to be a reduced level of the hormone, estrogen. This occurs after menopause in women, causing a rapid decline in bone mass over the next few years.

More recently, there has been some fear among young female athletes who either stop having periods or fail to start them at all. These conditions are also associated with reduced estrogen levels, and as a consequence bone mass can be lost at a time when young women should be laying down bone structure for the rest of their lives. While this may mean a higher risk of osteoporosis in older age, some sportswomen may also pay an immediate penalty in the form of an increased risk of stress fractures.

Other factors that increase the risk of loss of bone calcium are a poor intake of calcium in the diet, and excessive intake of salt and protein. Optimal training nutrition has already taken care of these last two items, so now it remains for us to protect bone structure with a healthy intake of calcium. A good target is as follows:

| | |
|---|---|
| Growing males (12–18 yrs) | 1000–1200mg calcium per day |
| Growing females (12–15 yrs) | 1000mg calcium per day |
| Adult males and females | 800mg calcium per day |
| Pregnancy (trimester 3) | 1100mg calcium per day |
| Breast-feeding | 1200mg calcium per day |
| Post-menopausal women | 1000mg calcium per day |
| Amenorrheic athletes | 1000mg calcium per day |

Table 2.8 provides a list of calcium-rich foods which fit into the high-carbohydrate or low-fat goals of the peak training diet. We are still awaiting a decision about the use of calcium supplements, but it is likely that the best calcium sources are found in foods.

**Table 2.8   Calcium-rich foods for the optimal training diet**

| Food | Serving | mg Calcium |
| --- | --- | --- |
| Skim milk | 200ml (glass) | 250mg |
| Low fat (1–2%) milk (Calcium added) | 200ml (glass) | 285mg |
| Reduced-fat cheese (11% fat slices) | 20g (1 slice) | 160mg |
| Cottage cheese | 100g (1/2 cup) | 80mg |
| Non-fat fruit yoghurt | 200g (carton) | 350mg |
| Low-fat icecream | 60g (2 Tbsp) | 90mg |
| Salmon (with bones) | 100g (small tin) | 335mg |
| Sardines (oil drained) | 100g (drained weight) | 380mg |
| Oysters | 100g | 135mg |
| Almonds | 50g | 125mg |
| Tahini | 20g (Tbsp) | 190mg |
| Spinach (cooked) | 145g (1 cup) | 72mg |
| Soy milk | 200ml (glass) | 45mg |
| Fortified soy milks (e.g. So Good) | 200ml (glass) | 290mg |
| Tofu | 100g | 130mg |

*Source*:   NUTTAB 1990, Australian Department of Community Services and Health

## 2.7   Timing of meals

Being an athlete probably means having a hectic lifestyle. Your daily schedule may include work or school, training (or competition), perhaps some physio or a massage, adequate sleep—and who knows what other commitments. Somewhere among all these activities, food has to be squeezed in, and unfortunately it often becomes an after-thought.

Your optimal training diet needs to be planned rather than haphazard. This way you will be sure that you are achieving all your nutrition goals. In addition, the timing of food can be an important factor in making it all happen—matching your food intake to the times when your body most appreciates it.

Your daily timetable and your commitments will be unique. Write down how you organise your schedule of events each day, and then take note of the following factors to see how you can best plot in your food stops over the day.

## HINTS FOR MEAL TIMING

- Spread the same food intake over five or six meals and snacks, rather than three large meals. The possible advantages are:

  - more even blood glucose levels rather than big peaks and troughs over the day. This may promote better glycogen synthesis and avoid 'flat spots' or afternoon fatigue.

  - lower blood fat levels and less likelihood of storing body fat for the same kilojoule load.

  - stimulation of your metabolic rate. Each time you eat a meal there is a small rise in your metabolic rate. More meals— better stimulation.

  - no need to 'stuff' yourself to eat lots of kilojoules. It is more comfortable to have a 'grazing' pattern—eat a little now and come back for more later.

  - avoids 'hunger spots' when you are on a reduced energy diet.

- Time your last meal before training (or competition) so that you can exercise comfortably. This may mean 1–2 hours for a light snack or a liquid meal (low-fat milk drink or Sustagen etc.) and up to 3–4 hours for larger or heavier meals.

- Promote recovery after heavy exercise sessions (training or competition) by eating some carbohydrate as soon as possible. Your high-carbohydrate breakfast or tea might be waiting for you as soon as you finish. If not, start muscle glycogen storage straight away with a carbohydrate drink or snack within 15–30 minutes of exercise, and continue to top up carbohydrate levels at your next meal. Don't neglect your fluid needs either. (Read Chapter 6 for more details on strategies to promote recovery.)

- Having access to food when you need it will be an important factor in achieving your nutrition goals. If you live your life on the run, you will need to plan ahead. Having a portable food supply with you will help you to eat on the go. Think of some suitable snacks to store at work, in your locker, in your sports bag or in your car.

# 3 Matters of physique—losing and gaining

While watching an Olympic Games parade, you may have noticed that athletes come in all shapes and sizes. You may also have tried to guess what type of sport was involved by examining the size and shape of a particular athlete. The issue at point is that various aspects of exercise performance are favoured by certain physical characteristics. Athletes, particularly at the highest level of play, will tend towards the physique that favours the demands of their sport.

Your physique will reflect both the basic structure you inherited from your parents, and the remoulding achieved by your training and diet. Hopefully you have chosen your parents well and selected the sport to which you are best suited! Physical characteristics that you may need to fine-tune are:

- your body-fat level
- your total muscle mass.

## 3.1 Desirable body-fat levels

We require a certain minimum level of body fat for good health. For men this is approximately 3–5 per cent of body weight, and for women about 12–15 per cent. Of course, most people carry considerably more body fat than this. In terms of sports performance, extra body fat can improve floatation, provide insulation against the cold, and protect body organs against damage during contact sports. However, these benefits must be weighed up against the extra weight of 'dead tissue' that must be carried. Extra body fat causes a decrease in your ratio of active to inactive body weight—often referred to as your power to weight ratio.

Some sports will not be disadvantaged by a higher level of body fat, particularly those based on skill rather than aerobic fitness. Think of golf or archery perhaps. By contrast, a low level of body fat is crucial for athletes such as triathletes and marathon runners, who must carry their own body weight over long distances. Similarly, athletes who compete in weight divisions will be better off if muscle is at a maximum level, and body fat is sacrificed to reach a weight limit.

In another set of sports again, success is partly or solely based on the athlete's appearance. Body builders, gymnasts and even divers pursue a 'trim, taut and terrific' look to impress the judges in their sports.

Typical body-fat levels for various sports have been compiled by taking measurements from large groups of elite athletes. This work is not meant to provide compulsory body-fat targets for each type of athlete. Rather, it should be used to describe a range of body-fat levels that appear *acceptable* or *desirable* for the top participants in a sport.

Within this range, athletes can probably find their own ideal body-fat level, based on the following information:

- at what body-fat level do you seem to perform best?
- can you also maintain good health at this level?
- can you achieve and maintain this body-fat level without unreasonable effort, and without compromising other nutritional goals?

Be aware that some athletes will perform at a top level, or at their personal best, at body-fat levels that fall outside the acceptable ranges. But then some top athletes don't fit the expected moulds in lots of ways—you probably know of very tall marathon runners or very short basketball players. And before you pursue the lowest level of body fat possible, be aware that too little body fat has its problems also. Athletes who become too lean can experience early fatigue, an increased risk of infection, intolerance to cold, and for some females, the loss of regular periods. There may be other penalties to pay, directly resulting from the methods used to achieve such a low body-fat level, such as drastic dieting or excessive training. So be sensible with your body-fat goals.

### 3.2 Assessment of body fat

There are a number of high-tech methods of estimating an athlete's body fat. Underwater weighing remains the golden standard, although like many methods it is expensive, belongs in a laboratory, and is generally only available to a few athletes. Even with the latest equipment and tightest techniques, no method is completely accurate. The results, usually given as the percentage of body fat in total body weight (% body fat), should always be interpreted with this in mind.

The ideal method would be portable, inexpensive and accessible to all athletes, without sacrificing its accuracy. The **pinch test**, with skinfold calipers being used to measure the fat under the skin at various body sites, has long provided a simple alternative. Traditionally, subcutaneous fat is measured at three or four sites and a prediction equation used to convert the results into an estimation of total body-fat content. This conversion step has always been regarded with suspicion, however, since it is impossible to find an equation that perfectly measures the relationship between skinfold fat and total body fat.

The Australian Institute of Sport has taken another approach to the skinfold exercise by doing away with the conversion step, and collecting new standards in terms of the skinfold measurements themselves—or at least their total sum. As this data bank of the 'sum of skinfolds' continues to grow, we should be able to set desirable ranges for many more sports and become better at interpreting the results.

The key points to this method are:

- A larger number of sites have been chosen to better represent body-fat distribution over the whole body. (See Figure 3.1 for a description of the sites—eight for males and seven for women.)

- Skinfold measurements should be taken by an experienced caliper technician using a good set of calipers (for example, John Bull or Harpenden calipers). Readings should be made on the right-hand side of the body, and after each site has been measured once, the whole sequence should be repeated. Where the second reading differs by more than 0.5mm, a third measurement should be taken. The average of the two closest values is used.

- The sum of the eight or seven skinfold readings is then calculated. This can be compared to the 'sum of skinfold' standards for the particular sport, or, better still, to previous measurements made on the same athlete.

- If an athlete has skinfold measurements repeated over a period of time to monitor changes, it is preferable that the same technician takes the readings on each occasion.

Typical readings for the sum of skinfolds will be presented for various sports in Part II of this book.

### 3.3 Losing body fat

So your lycra outfit is showing bulges in the wrong places or perhaps you have come back from injury to find that your skinfold sum has jumped by 20mm. Maybe you need to lose 3kg to row in the light-weight crew. At some point in their lives or their sporting careers, most people try to lose weight.

The real aim is not to lose weight but to lose body fat, and this is achieved by consistently eating less kilojoules than your body expends, thus creating an energy loss situation. This might sound simple,

**Figure 3.1  Sites for taking skinfold (fat) measurements for determination of skinfold sum**

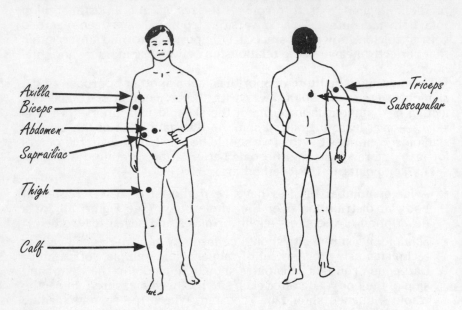

Triceps — *vertical skinfold on the back of the arm, midway between shoulder and elbow processes*

Biceps — *vertical skinfold on the front of the arm, midway between shoulder and elbow processes*

Axilla — *(males only) vertical skinfold taken on the 'under arm' line with subject placing his hand on his head*

Subscapular — *oblique skinfold taken about 1cm below the scapula (shoulder blade)*

Abdomen — *vertical skinfold taken next to the navel*

Suprailiac — *oblique skinfold taken 4cm above the hip bone (iliac crest)*

Thigh — *vertical skinfold taken on front of leg halfway between hip bone and knee cap*

Calf — *vertical skinfold taken on inside of lower leg at its greatest circumference, subject seated.*

**Table 3.1   Keys to a healthy fat-loss program for athletes**

1   Goals: Set realistic weight loss goals, including short-term targets and a long-term aim.
2   Time frame: Plan to lose 0.5 to 1.0kg each week. This may not happen in a consistent and consecutive way, but can be used as an overall timeline.
3   Energy intake: Plan to shed about 2000–4000 kilojoules from your daily requirements (500–1000 Cals). More than this and you may cause a metabolic adjustment.
4   Carbohydrate intake: Make sure that you can still eat adequate carbohydrate intake for training, or you will quickly become fatigued.
5   Protein intake: Are you meeting your daily requirements?
6   Vitamins and minerals: Your health and performance will suffer if you become nutritionally depleted. You will need to be clever with food choices to maintain your daily needs. A dietitian may suggest an additional supplement.
7   Flexibility: Does your eating plan fit in with your daily schedule?
8   Long-term: Can you see yourself maintaining these eating habits as long as you want to maintain your fat-loss goals?
9   Enjoyment: Make sure that some of your favourite foods can be fitted into the plan—perhaps for special occasions and in small amounts.

but in actual practice, the weight loss attempts of most people end in failure. Instead of simple and consistent means, some athletes seek a magical program that will require no effort and produce results by last Thursday. Some turn to grapefruit diets, herbal powders or 'fat burning' supplements. Others take drastic measures such as severe food restriction, dehydration techniques, diuretics and laxatives.

Since these methods fail to address either energy loss or long-term issues, they also fail to produce the desired fat loss. In addition, some attempts will actually depress the body's metabolic rate, making it even more difficult to create an energy loss situation. In the worst case scenario, there may be direct effects on your exercise performance or your health. While some people make a life-time career of being on (and off) diets, there is only one successful way to approach weight loss—and that's once and for all!

The first step is to forget the magic and miracles, and to be prepared to invest a little effort and sufficient time. The time element is essential. To lose 1kg of body fat, you must create an energy loss of almost 30 000 kilojoules (7000 Calories). Since most people can only afford to spare 2000–4000 kilojoules per day (500–1000 Calories), you will need 7–14 days to burn up one kg of body fat. On the bright side, once it is gone, it is gone—unless you revert back to your old food habits and put yourself into a energy gain situation.

What is the formula for the peak nutrition fat-loss diet? Table 3.1 summarises the key features that you should plan to incorporate, with realistic goals and adequate time being first on the list. It is best not to juggle weight loss and a competition schedule. Plan to tackle it early in training or even in the off-season. By protecting your intake of important nutrients, you should be able to continue training without fear of fatigue caused by dietary deficiencies.

Such a diet can come from a dietitian or a good sports nutrition book. Depending on your present energy requirements you may need a 8400 kJ (2000 Cal), 10 500 kJ (2500 Cal) or even 12 600 kJ (3000 Cal) daily food plan.

Another approach to body-fat loss is to remodel your present diet, which probably already meets some of the goals of a peak nutrition fat-loss plan. For a start you probably enjoy what you eat and it fits your lifestyle. So take a good look at your present eating patterns and decide where some cost-cutting can be done to reduce total energy intake, while preserving your other nutritional goals. A dietitian is an expert at this exercise, but you may be able to plan some changes by yourself.

Of course, make sure that you work with a realistic picture of what you actually eat, rather than what you think you eat. A helpful way to sort this out is to keep a food record for a week, writing down everything that you eat or drink at the time it happens. Additional comments about why you ate (or drank) these items can help you to find the right strategies to make changes.

You may need to work on three basic issues of eating: the quantity you eat, the type of food you eat, and your reasons for eating. You will need to make permanent changes to your eating patterns along these lines and check periodically, by keeping another record, to see that the effort is sustained.

### 3.4  Low-energy consumers

Some athletes seem to defy energy logic. Many need to drop to very low kilojoule intakes, even below 6400 kJ/day (1500 Cals), to lose body fat. Some seem to exist on these low levels just to maintain their body weight. For years this phenomenon has puzzled nutritionists

---

**HINTS FOR SUCCESSFUL AND SUSTAINED LOSS OF BODY FAT**

*Quantity of food*

- Decide exactly how much you *need* to eat, as distinct from what you would *like* to eat or what everyone else is eating. This may mean reducing your usual serve by a half or a third, and stopping yourself from going back for seconds.

- Avoid letting yourself get too hungry before you eat. A small but well-timed snack may prevent you from eating everything in sight later on.

- Eat slowly so that you enjoy your food and can stop before you overeat.
- Make your meals as filling as possible:
  - — drink water (or a low-kilojoule drink) before and during your meal
  - — enjoy high-fibre foods
- Eat fruit rather than drink juice. Take care with all high-energy fluids—it is easy to quaff litres of kilojoules, especially when you are thirsty after training!
- Enjoy your special or favourite foods, but in smaller quantities. For example, share a dessert in a restaurant, or have a chocolate frog rather than a family block.

*Type of food*

- Target fat, alcohol and sugar in your diet. These are high-energy nutrients that contribute little nutrient value to your diet (see Chapter 1 for more details).

*Eating behaviour*

From your food record, take note of the reasons that you eat without being hungry or really needing the food. Stop the eating by changing your behaviour, for example:

- Eating when depressed or upset—tackle the problem that is causing you to be depressed or upset. Think up other activities to pamper yourself that don't involve food.
- Eating when bored—find a non-food activity, as above.
- Eating because the food is around—either remove yourself or re-move the food. There is no such thing as willpower!
- Eating at social functions—at a restaurant, order exactly what you want and don't be afraid to make special requests. Eat just what you want and don't be afraid to say 'no thank you' to your hosts. Better still, ring your hosts ahead of time and explain what you need. As a last option, don't eat at all (eat before you go, or when you get home).
- Find non-food ways of rewarding yourself for successful changes in your food habits.

and athletes alike. Some have refused to believe that it actually happens, claiming that these athletes under-report the food that they eat.

While this may be true to some extent and for some athletes, there is a definite group who are low-energy consumers. We might define this as any male athlete who chronically eats less than 8400 kJ per day (2000 Cals) and any female athlete who chronically eats less than 6400 kJ per day (1500 Cals). Likely candidates for the low-energy group are athletes who strive to be petite and lean, but whose training is skill-based rather than energy burning—gymnasts and ballet dancers for example. Another group are the chronic dieters who have gradually lowered their metabolic rate by years of restricting energy intake. Female athletes of all types, as well as athletes who 'make weight' might be nominated in this group.

These athletes are set enormous challenges to achieve their nutrient requirements from such a small energy budget. The features of the peak nutrition fat-loss plan (Table 3.1) are still important here. To these we might add the following ideas:

---

### HINTS FOR LOW-ENERGY CONSUMERS

- Look at ways of increasing your energy requirements, either by increasing the cost of energy for exercise, or by increasing/preserving metabolic rate:

    — if your program consists of skill- or strength-training only it may be possible to add some aerobic activities to increase the total energy cost of your training. Talk to your coach about this.

    — Even on a fat-loss program, do not drop below a daily intake of 5000 kJ (1200 Cals) for females and 7600 kJ (1800 Cals) for males. Further restrictions probably promote metabolic conservation, and make nutrient intake goals almost impossible.

    — Spread your energy intake over the day. Do not skip meals—especially breakfast—if you want to preserve your metabolic rate.

- You will need to work hard to achieve maximum nutrient intake from minimum kilojoules:

    — consult a dietitian to learn how to match your needs to clever food use

    — you will probably need to take a nutrient supplement to add to your food intake. A dietitian can advise you on the best type and the right dose.

---

## 3.5 Making weight

Weight-matched sports include boxing, wrestling, judo, weight- and power-lifting, horse racing and lightweight rowing. There are two traditions in these sports that show the nastier side of athletic nutritional practices. The first is the desire to compete in a lower weight division than your normal training weight—theoretically gaining an advantage over a lighter, weaker opponent.

The second tradition is to shed the excess weight in a rapid fashion—often three to six kilos in as many days. This is when the drastic techniques come into play—such as dehydrating in saunas or plastic suits, fasting, or using diuretics and laxatives. These methods may effectively cause a loss of body weight, but the athlete loses body water, muscle and glycogen stores to achieve it. Are you prepared for the loss of performance and the health hazards involved? Even if you have time for a meal after the weigh-in, cramming yourself with food and drink cannot quickly reverse the damage.

Clearly, there needs to be a radical change of thinking and practice in these sports. The bottom line? You will compete best at the weight that corresponds to your lowest healthy body-fat level. Achieve this once and for all, and leave yourself only minor adjustments of one or two kg before an event. With pre-competition nerves and a few last minute tricks, you should be able to weigh-in confidently and in peak form.

## 3.6 Bulking-up

Many athletes, even outside bodybuilding, dream of looking like Arnold Schwarzenegger. Often they try to buy these dreams with pills, potions, powders and three helpings at each meal. But it is not pure weight gain that is desired. Athletes in strength-based sports such as throwing events, power- and weight-lifting, and some football codes, are really after a gain in muscle mass. Despite all the magic and misconceptions, there are only a few real requirements for muscle gain, and these, in order of importance are:

- genetic potential—did you pick the right parents with the right body type?
- weight training—muscles only grow when given the right stimulation.
- a high-energy diet—you need more of everything, including, but not exclusively, a high protein intake. In fact, carbohydrate is still the most important energy source, since the muscle must be fuelled to do the work that will stimulate it to grow.

Set realistic goals based on the first two points in this list. You may need to seek expert advice—a strength coach to set a program of

---

HINTS FOR 'MAKING WEIGHT'

- Select a competition weight that is safe and sensible, by assessing your lowest healthy body-fat level. Use the fat-loss methods above to slowly and surely achieve this weight, well ahead of your competition.
- Stay within one or two kilos of your weight division during training.
- Final adjustments might be made over the last week to ten days with a further slight reduction in energy intake—especially if you are in an exercise taper.
- Over the last week, reduce salt intake and stay away from high-salt foods to prevent fluid retention.
- To lose the final kilogram, make use of a low-residue diet over the last 12–24 hours. The easiest plan is to replace meals with liquid meal supplements like Exceed Sports Nutrition Supplement and Sustagen. These supplements will supply carbohydrate for muscle stores and other nutrients, but leave your gut empty and light.
- Leave your pre-event meal until after the weigh-in. This doesn't need to be a huge feast, but should top up your energy and fluid levels before the event.

---

progressive muscle overload, and a dietitian to support this with a high-energy diet. Periodic measurement of body-fat levels and muscle circumferences will reassure you that any resulting gains in body weight are those that are desired.

### 3.7 The high-energy diet

Whether you are trying to gain muscle mass or simply maintain a strenuous training load, you may need to consume a large daily energy intake. To outsiders this may sound like paradise—and for some it *can* be enjoyable. But for other athletes it can range from a chore to an impossible task. Hurdles to chewing through all the necessary kilojoules include:

- lack of time, including time to buy and prepare food. Subtract your training time, your work, sleep and all the other commitments in your day, and this probably leaves you with three hours to consume 25 000 kilojoules (6000 Cals).
- the bulk of the food. A high-carbohydrate, high-fibre diet mean lots to chew and digest.
- fatigue and loss of appetite after training.

- lack of access to food (or suitable food) at possible eating times.
- need to limit food intake prior to training to avoid gastrointestinal discomfort during exercise.

If you are having trouble, a dietitian can help you to look over the day's schedule of activities. Keep a record like that suggested in the fat-loss section. This will help you look for opportunities to increase your energy intake.

---

## HINTS FOR ACHIEVING A HIGH-ENERGY INTAKE

- Above all, be organised. You will need to apply the same dedication to your eating program that you apply to your training. A haphazard approach—eating what is available, when it is convenient—is no way to ensure the quality and quantity of food that you need.
- Increase the number of times you eat rather than the size of meals. A 'grazing' pattern of six to eight meals and snacks enables greater intake and circumvents gastric discomfort compared to the conventional pattern of three large meals. Build this into your day to suit your schedule.
- Plan to have food on hand for every eating opportunity. Portable snacks may be useful and an emergency food supply in your car, sports bag or locker is another good idea.
- Increase the energy content of high-carbohydrate foods by adding a little sugar or low-fat protein. For example, add jams and syrups to toast and pancakes, and make two or three layer fillings in sandwiches. This adds extra kilojoules to a nutritious meal, without adding bulk.
- Avoid excessive intake of fibre, and make use of some 'white' cereal foods with less bulk (e.g. white bread, Cornflakes and Rice Bubbles). You may find it impossible to chew your way through a diet that is solely based on wholegrain and high-fibre foods.
- Drink high-energy fluids. Make low-fat milkshakes and fruit smoothies, or try liquid meal supplements such as Exceed Sports Nutrition Supplement or Sustagen. These drinks provide low-bulk nutritious kilojoules and can be consumed with meals or as snacks between meals—even quite close to training.

---

# 4 Competition nutrition

Competition is your time to 'seize the day' and push yourself beyond your best. Your training and tapering should leave you well prepared for this. The final detail to consider is what could go wrong, to acknowledge the physiological issues that might hold you back, and then to plot nutritional strategies to keep these problems at bay. Each type of sport will have its own 'walls' to hit—whether it be lactate accumulation, muscle fuel exhaustion, or dehydration. Your nutritional strategies will involve issues of preparation over the last days as well as special practices during the competition itself.

## 4.1 A checklist of fatigue factors

The fatigue factors in a sport relate mostly to the type and duration of exercise involved. But the environment also can add to the problem list.

In brief, for explosive efforts such as jumps and lifts, fuel is supplied by high-energy phosphate compounds within the muscle cell—adenosine triphosphate (ATP) and creatine phosphate. These compounds can only supply several seconds of work but are quickly generated between efforts. Unless you have drastically starved or dehydrated yourself to get to the event there is probably little else that can reduce your physical potential. So go for it!

As events move from seconds to minutes, still at high workloads, metabolism continues anaerobically (without oxygen) with muscle glycogen now providing the main fuel source. If you start the event with extremely low levels you will be without a fuel source. But more likely, your normal muscle glycogen stores will see you through and it will be the build-up of lactic acid and other by-products of muscle metabolism that cause the burning fatigue that slows you.

As the exercise duration becomes longer—and therefore at a lower intensity—aerobic metabolism becomes more important. Your muscles burn a fuel concoction of fat and carbohydrate, with the relative proportion of each depending on factors including the intensity of exercise (the carbohydrate contribution is greater at a higher workload) and your level of training.

Team sports usually involve a mixture of (anaerobic) high intensity bursts, interspersed with (aerobic) recovery periods. Meanwhile, athletes in relatively steady-state exercise, such as running or cycling, will gravitate to a predominantly aerobic workload just below the threshold where lactate accumulation causes fatigue. Both groups should be able to continue activity until carbohydrate fuel stores become depleted.

The failure of carbohydrate stores to keep pace with the energy demands of the muscle occurs typically after 60–90 minutes of continuous exercise at maximal aerobic pace. Fatigue can be manifested in two ways, known by runners as 'hitting the wall' or in cyclists' and triathletes' terms, as 'bonking'. The 'wall' describes local muscle fatigue—heaviness or cramping in the exercising muscle—causing the athlete to slow down, and sometimes even stop completely. The likely cause is the exhaustion of muscle glycogen stores, leaving the muscle to rely on fat and the uptake of glucose from the blood stream to supply energy.

'Bonking' is caused primarily by the lowering of blood glucose levels, and occurs when the muscles take up blood glucose more quickly than it can be replaced by the liver (or by eating/drinking carbohydrate). This often happens in conjunction with muscle glycogen depletion, but in some sensitive individuals it may occur as an independent event. 'Bonking' produces a central nervous system fatigue—dizziness and mental confusion, and an overwhelming tiredness and desire to sleep. The smart athlete will try to avoid both consequences of carbohydrate depletion.

Dehydration is a fatigue factor in many sports, with as little as 2–4 per cent body fluid loss (1–2kg for a 50kg athlete and 1.5–3kg for a 75kg athlete) being shown to cause a reduction in aerobic exercise output. When fluid losses move into the range of 5–10 per cent of body weight, heat exhaustion may become a threat—although heat-related problems also present separately without dehydration.

Dehydration can occur in sport from two angles. Firstly some athletes purposely dehydrate themselves before an event to make a weight category. Talk about starting the event behind the eight ball! Secondly, dehydration can occur during exercise as athletes fail to replace the sweat losses that occur to cool their bodies. Just like a car, you produce heat as a by-product of work and this must be dissipated to keep your body at its preferred temperature. The harder you work and the heavier you are, the more sweat will be produced to cool you down. If the environmental temperature is hot and humid, your body will find it difficult to dissipate this heat.

The final nutritionally-based fatigue factor is a blood sodium imbalance. This is really only an issue for athletes who exercise at high intensities for very long periods—perhaps six hours or more—especially in the heat. Athletes such as ultradistance runners and Ironman triathletes actually do this! In recent years it has been found that many of these athletes finish with low blood-sodium levels, and a small percentage suffer severe effects as a result. Although the exact reason for diluted blood sodium levels is still debated, it is likely that problems arise when large amounts of sweat (fluid and sodium) are replaced with large amounts of low-sodium fluids such as water or cold drinks. There is a suggestion that a few athletes overdrink as well as choose their fluids poorly.

The message here is that you should drink to keep pace with your sweat rate—neither greatly underestimating nor drinking more than you are losing. While it is rare, it is possible for an athlete who is moving slowly—perhaps at the rear of the field—to spend too much time at the aid stations and outdrink gentle sweat losses. As for the choice of beverage, a sports drink containing electrolytes may better assist in maintaining blood volume and contents during situations of prolonged exercise.

### 4.2  General preparation for competition

Your checklist for competition preparation should include the following items:

- ensure that fuel stores (glycogen) are topped up in both your muscles and liver to meet the demands of your particular sport;
- in weight-class sports, achieve the required body weight without sacrificing performance;
- be well-hydrated;
- avoid gastrointestinal discomfort or problems;
- eat a pre-event meal that will continue to meet these goals.

Making weight to reach a competition weight class has already been discussed in Chapter 3.5. This leaves fuel and fluid needs as your preparation priorities on the day(s) leading up to the event. How hard you need to prepare depends on the challenges of your sport, the importance of the event and the frequency of competition. A long, intense event will probably throw out more fatigue factors to battle against, and if this your major competition for the year then you will want to leave nothing to chance.

In preparing your fuel stores for competition, you can rest a little easier knowing that your training has given you an edge in this department. Aerobic endurance training teaches your muscles to store greater amounts of glycogen and to use it more sparingly during aerobic exercise, by increasing the contribution of fat to the fuel mixture. With your everyday (increased) muscle glycogen stores intact at the beginning of an event, you will have enough fuel on board to see you through all but the most prolonged sporting events.

HINTS FOR PREPARATION FOR GENERAL SPORTS
COMPETITION (events up to 80 minutes of
continuous exercise)

- In the absence of muscle damage, 24–36 hours of rest and a high carbohydrate diet will allow the storage of adequate muscle glycogen to see you through the event. For some athletes the only change will be a well-earned rest from training.

- If you are competing frequently—once or twice a week for example, you may not always be able to organise the required rest from exercise. Try to taper exercise and achieve better preparation for your most important events.

- Schedule training so that the sessions which could potentially damage muscle fibres, (for example, those involving hard running, body contact or eccentric weight work) are early in the week, allowing more time for recovery.

- Your everyday training diet should already be high in carbohydrate. However, you may like to use the carbohydrate ready reckoner (Table 2.4) to check that your diet provides 9–10g of carbohydrate for every kilogram you weigh. For example, a 50kg athlete should aim to eat 450–500g of carbohydrate over the day preceding competition, while a 80kg athlete might aim for 700–800g of carbohydrate.

- If extra carbohydrate is needed over your everyday patterns, you might need to accentuate carbohydrate foods and reduce the protein component of meals. A little extra sugar and sugary foods can provide some compact carbohydrate—but don't make this an excuse to eat lots of fat.

- Drink plenty of fluids—especially if you anticipate that you will be competing in a hot environment.

- Top off with a good pre-event meal (see section 4.4).

To reach this everyday potential for muscle glycogen storage you require:

- 24–36 hours of rest or tapered exercise
- daily intake of at least 9–10g of carbohydrate per kilogram of your body weight
- absence of muscle damage.

For many athletes these conditions might be met simply by combining their everyday high-carbohydrate diet with a rest from training.

Athletes in sports in which frequent competitions require more frequent preparation will need to plan carefully and prioritise their events. Notice in the hints on the previous page, that there is no need to cram yourself with food like this is your last meal.

### 4.3  Carbohydrate loading for endurance events

Carbohydrate loading is probably the most talked about, yet least understood, nutrition topic in sport. For a start, all athletes, from darts players to a ultramarathon runner think they need to do it. Secondly, many athletes use carbo-loading as a euphemism for gluttony—never mind the quality of the food, make up for it with quantity. And finally, the technique has been refined since its birth in the 1960s, but many athletes have yet to catch up with the news.

To sort out the mysticism from what is a potentially valuable practice, you should firstly decide whether your sport requires you to have super-loaded muscle glycogen stores. If you are going to drive around the block, you don't need to have an extra petrol tank in your car—it would just be extra weight to carry. However, if you are driving in an endurance rally, then you will have an opportunity to use the additional fuel.

Typically, endurance sports which involve over 90 minutes of continuous high-intensity exercise, using the same muscle groups, will challenge the capacity of the athlete's normal fuel stores. Think about this definition carefully. Although your triathlon may take over two hours, it involves three separate sports and therefore different muscle groups. And while a team game may also play out this time, the actual duration of activity performed by any one player may be considerably shorter. You may need to think back to past events—did your pace or performance drop off late in the competition, accompanied by symptoms of muscle glycogen fatigue? If so, then you may be helped by super-loading muscle glycogen stores before you start. You won't run faster or work harder in the beginning, but it will prolong the time that you can exercise at your optimum pace. In the long run, you will come out on top.

Once you have decided that you compete in an endurance sport and that carbohydrate loading could be useful, the next step is to forget everything you have read or heard about it—particularly about depletion phases and low carbohydrate diets. In its place try the following modified—and simplified—technique.

Without going into great detail, the original or classical carbohydrate loading program familiar to most athletes was developed using healthy but essentially non-elite subjects. We now know that well-trained endurance athletes are 'lean, mean glycogen-storing machines'. Every day in training they use up large amounts of glycogen, and every day their muscles toil to rebuild the stores. In fact, this is a continuous

**Figure 4.1  The 'modified' carbo - loading program**

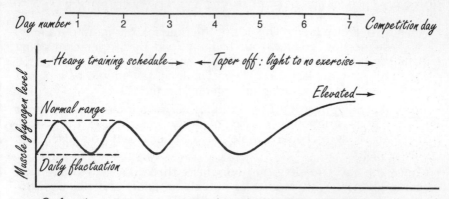

*Daily endurance training causes a daily cycle of depletion and loading of muscle glycogen stores. 72 hours of rest/taper and a high carbohydrate intake (10g/kg body weight per day) will cause an 'overloading' of glycogen in the trained muscles, enabling competition performance to continue for a longer period at an optimal pace.*

mini-cycle of depleting and loading. With the storage techniques already well-rehearsed, all a well-trained athlete has to do to load up their muscle glycogen stores is to give their muscles the luxury of more time.

The same conditions needed for general competition preparation apply to modified carbohydrate loading, except that for a full glycogen storage effect you must extend the exercise taper and high-carbohydrate diet to a 72-hour period. Figure 4.1 illustrates how muscles become glycogen-loaded simply by extending the general preparation technique over a longer time. It is unlikely that you will compete in a true endurance event on a weekly basis, but if you do, save the full 72-hour preparation for important events only. As long as the taper doesn't interfere with your training schedule you can carbo-load, using this modified program, as often as necessary.

### 4.4  The pre-event meal

Presuming that your competition preparation has already organised full muscle glycogen stores, the major goals of the pre-event meal are:

- to top-up liver glycogen stores, especially if you are competing in the morning;
- to top-up fluid levels;

63

HINTS FOR A 'MODIFIED' CARBOHYDRATE LOADING PROGRAM

- Plan an exercise taper. This is not the time for last-minute training. As a suggestion, reduce your training load by 50 per cent going into the last week before the event, and reduce it by another 50 per cent over the last three days. The final day should be a day of rest—use it for stretching and mental preparation.

- Your daily diet over the 72-hour taper period should provide about 9–10g of carbohydrate per kg of body weight. Use the carbohydrate ready reckoner (Table 2.4) to check that you reach this daily target.

- Since the carbo-loading diet only lasts three days, you may take some liberties with your total nutritional goals and place carbohydrate intake at the top of the list. For example, don't worry about the protein foods at your meals—by de-emphasising the serve, you can leave yourself more room for large serves of the carbohydrate foods. In addition, sugar and sugary foods, including drinks such as sports drinks and soft drinks, can provide a compact carbohydrate source. Table 4.1 provides a typical carbo-loading menu.

- Be extra careful with your fat intake—save the kilojoules for carbohydrates. Don't get tricked with high-fat carbohydrate foods such as chocolate, icecream, rich desserts and takeaways. Although favourites with many carbo-loading athletes, these foods are a rich source of fat rather than carbohydrate.

- Enjoy the official carbo-loading functions before your event but don't let yourself get carried away. Leave your competitiveness for the event, not for food consumption races. Hopefully the event organisers have enlisted the aid of a dietitian in devising the menu, so the food will be suitable. Again, don't end up fat-loading instead of carbo-loading.

- Over the final 24 hours you may wish to reduce your gastric contents so that you race feeling light. To do this, switch to low-fibre foods and make extra use of compact sugar foods. You may even like to use a combination of liquid meal supplements (Sustagen or Exceed Sports Nutrition Supplement) or the high-carbohydrate carbo-loader supplements to supply some or all of your carbohydrate needs over the last 12–24 hours. These are very low in residue and will leave you with an empty gut to race light.

- Drink plenty of fluids, as your muscles will store water along with the glycogen. You will need to be well-hydrated for a long event, especially in hot weather. Perhaps carry a water bottle around with you over the last 24 hours as a reminder.

• Finish up with a light pre-event meal two to three hours prior to the event (see Section 4.4)—and compete with action-packed muscles!

**Table 4.1  A typical plan for carbohydrate loading**

*These meal plans provide about 600g of carbohydrate per day-suitable for a 60 kg athlete to meet the 10g/kg recommendations. You may need to adapt the menus to eat more or less carbohydrate.*

*The menus are proposed for carbohydrate loading days only—while meeting carbohydrate requirements, they do not meet all nutritional goals for everyday eating.*

**Day 1**: (602g CHO, 80 per cent of energy intake—12 200 kJ)
| | |
|---|---|
| Breakfast: | 2 cups Weeties + 1 cup skim milk |
| | 1 cup sweetened canned peaches |
| | 250ml sweetened fruit juice |
| Snack: | 2 slices thick toast + scrape marg + Tbsp honey |
| | 250ml sports drink |
| Lunch: | 2 large bread rolls with light salad |
| | 375ml can soft drink |
| Snack: | Large coffee scroll (unbuttered) |
| | 250ml fruit juice |
| Dinner: | 3 cups of boiled rice |
| | (made into light stir fry  with small amount of lean ham, peas, corn and onion) |
| | 250ml fruit juice |
| Snack: | 2 crumpets + scrape marg + Tbsp jam |
| | Tea/coffee |
| Extra water during day | |

**Day 2**: (605g CHO, 77 per cent of energy, 12 700 kJ)
| | |
|---|---|
| Breakfast: | 2 cups porridge + 1 cup skim milk |
| | 1 banana |
| | 250ml sweetened fruit juice |
| Snack: | 2 muffins + scrape marg + Tbsp jam |
| Lunch: | Stack of three pancakes + 60ml of maple syrup + small scoop icecream |
| | 250ml fruit juice |
| Snack: | 50g jelly beans |
| Dinner: | 3 cups cooked pasta + 1 cup tomato puree |
| | 2 slices bread |
| | 250ml sports drink |
| Snack: | 1 cup fresh fruit salad |
| | 2 Tbsp non-fat flavoured yoghurt |

**Day 3**:
| | |
|---|---|
| same as Day 1 or 2, switching to white cereals, bread, etc. | |
| OR: | in place of lunch, dinner and afternoon/evening snacks: |
| | 500ml liquid meal or high carbohydrate supplement (carbo-loader) on each occasion (plus light snack if desired) |
| Extra water during day | |

- to fill the stomach to a point of comfort where you do not feel empty and hungry during the event, but nor do you suffer discomfort from overfilling or from gastrointestinal upsets;
- to leave you feeling confident and ready!

This is rather a mixed bag, since athletes vary with their food likes and dislikes, as well as the amount of food they consider comfortable. Since sport can be played at almost any time of the day, the pre-event meal schedule may vary considerably from one athlete to the next. When their event starts late in the day, some athletes simply continue to eat their normal daily meal pattern, until say, four hours pre-event. Others might like to eat larger meals in the early part of the day, and finish with a light snack up to two hours pre-event. In both cases, significant amounts of carbohydrate are eaten during the day to top-up glycogen stores.

Athletes who participate in morning competition may experiment with a larger meal three to four hours pre-event, or a small snack one or two hours pre-event. It is important that some food is eaten, even in very early morning events, since after an overnight fast your liver stores need to be topped up.

The psychological impact, and even superstition attached to favourite pre-event foods must also be considered. In many ways the pre-event meal is a just fine-tuning effect after all the important preparation work has been done. Even where pre-event meal practices don't exactly meet the scientific theories, some athletes will not be significantly disadvantaged. If the athlete is emotionally or psychologically boosted by a strategy, it is often best to leave well enough alone.

### 4.5   Sugar prior to the event?

In days past, some athletes thought that a last-minute intake of sugar might provide instant energy to boost their competition performance—hence the cramming of chocolate bars, glucose tablets and other foods thought of as quick energy. However, some of these foods are high-fat as well as high-carbohydrate. And more to the point, the most important carbohydrate source for muscle at the start of exercise is stored right inside it. That is why you carefully prepared your diet and taper over the day(s) leading up to this event.

The major effect of a large dose of sugar or glucose in the 30–60 minutes prior to exercise is to increase your carbohydrate metabolism, by increasing blood glucose and insulin levels. This is a bit like pulling out the choke on a car to make it burn a richer fuel. Some researchers have found that the increased carbohydrate burning continues on into the exercise bout, increasing the ratio of carbohydrate that is burnt in aerobic exercise at the expense of fat-burning.

HINTS FOR THE PRE-EVENT MEAL

- Plan your day so that the final meal is eaten four hours before the event in the case of a larger meal, or one to two hours pre-event in the case of a snack.

- Choose high-carbohydrate, low-fat foods to ensure easy digestion and to top up carbohydrate fuel supplies. Many people find their normal breakfast choices are a great pre-event meal, even when it is not breakfast time. Other ideas are found in 'Pre-event Meal Ideas'.

- Experiment with the type, timing and amount of food that works best for you. Practise in training or some minor competitions so that everything is right for important challenges. Learn which foods, if any, cause you discomfort or upsets and avoid these.

- Drink plenty of fluids leading up to the event. If it is a hot day, or your sport provides little opportunity to drink during the competition, make sure that you are well-hydrated at the start of the event.

- In sports where you must weigh-in prior to the event to meet a weight division, you will probably choose to leave your pre-event food and fluid intake until after the weigh-in. Check-in times can be early in the morning on the day of the event, or an hour before it starts. Hopefully you have used sensible weight control measures to reach your weight target, so your pre-event meal will only need to top up fuel and fluid stores. There should never be a need for a last-minute panic to cram in food. It is too late in the day to correct the effects of dehydration and starvation practices.

- If you suffer from competition nerves, you might find liquid meal supplements a useful pre-event meal—such as Sustagen or Exceed Sports Nutrition Supplement. These are high in carbohydrate and low in fat and bulk. Being easy to digest, you can probably drink them in comfort even up to an hour pre-event.

For an endurance athlete this might pose a problem, since body carbohydrate fuel stores will now be depleted at a faster rate. Other athletes may be sensitive to a lowering effect on blood glucose. However, other studies have shown that as soon as the exercise gets into full swing, metabolism reverts back to its normal pattern and no problems occur. In any case, it is generally advised that the consumption of large amounts of sugars within the last 30–60 minutes before exercise is unnecessary and to be avoided. Even if there are no metabolic disadvantages, some people will suffer diarrhea from such a large sugar load.

---

PRE-EVENT MEAL IDEAS

- Breakfast cereal + skim milk + fresh/canned fruit
- Muffins or crumpets + jam/honey
- Pancakes + syrup
- Toast + baked beans
- Baked potatoes with low-fat filling
- Creamed rice (made with skim milk)
- Spaghetti with tomato or low-fat sauce
- Rolls or sandwiches with banana filling
- Fruit salad plus low fat yoghurt
- Liquid meal (Sustagen or Exceed Sports Nutrition Supplement)

---

Athletes who compete in high-intensity anaerobic events lasting seconds to minutes are already big carbohydrate-burners. For these athletes, carbohydrate between and before events will be part of recovering between one heat or bout, and preparing for the next. Small carbohydrate snacks, including sugary foods, can be spread over the day of competition and will help to preserve blood glucose levels. Again, large doses of sugar are best avoided. All strategies should be practised in training and minor competitions so that any problems will be found out in advance.

### 4.6 Fluid intake during events

During any sport, it makes sense to stay as well-hydrated as possible. Even moderate fluid losses, probably unnoticed by most athletes, will impair performance levels, especially in hot conditions. You should aim to keep total fluid deficits below two to three per cent of body weight—probably 1–2kg for most athletes. During intense exercise, particularly in hot weather or in a closed environment, an athlete can lose up to one or two litres of sweat per hour. This means that in any sport with a duration of at least 60 minutes of continuous high-intensity exercise, there is a need to consider fluid levels.

In many cases the threat of dehydration can be removed, or at least reduced, by the provision of fluids to competitors during the event. While this is not always necessary or practical in every sport, as the environmental conditions become hotter and the duration of the sport increases, fluid intake during the event becomes more important. A healthy tradition in many sports is to have quarter-time or half-time

## HINTS FOR FLUID INTAKE DURING GENERAL SPORTS COMPETITION

- Events typically lasting for 50–60 minutes of continuous exercise should provide opportunities for fluid intake during competition. Depending on the nature of the sport you may need to organise aid stations, scheduled drink breaks, or the use of trainers/watercarriers to bring out drinks.

- Athletes who compete in brief, intense sports lasting seconds to minutes should rehydrate fully after events, especially where they intend to compete or train again later in the day.

- Athletes who are slightly dehydrated before a competition weigh-in, should work hard after the weigh-in to fully restore fluid levels. If the competition involves further sweating, such as a wrestling match or a rowing event, then extra care should be taken.

- Water is a suitable drink for most events, though sports drinks, and diluted (de-fizzed) soft drinks or cordials offer no real disadvantages other than their cost. Above all, a drink must taste good!

- Cold drinks are more refreshing and palatable.

- Try to drink regularly rather than waiting until you become thirsty, and drink a comfortable amount on each occasion—for example, 150–250ml.

- In some sports these fluid intake guidelines might clash with tradition, attitudes and sometimes even sports rules. There may be a need for re-education of athletes and re-organisation of event practices to transform these ideas into action. Athletes should appreciate that the concern over fluid balance is not just to prevent severe dehydration, but to promote optimum performance at all times.

drink stops, aid stations on the race route, or trainers armed with water-bottles waiting for a break in the game. Look at your sport to see whether the need arises and what opportunities can be provided for fluid intake.

Since the primary need is for fluid, the simplest and most practical drink is water. Interestingly, water does not provide the most rapid form of water replacement in the body. A dilute carbohydrate-electrolyte drink will actually deliver water faster to the body, since small amounts of glucose and sodium increase intestinal uptake of water. However, water still does the job and in general, in a non-endurance sport, fluid replacement needs although important, are usually moderate. If you don't mind paying the extra cost, then flavoured drinks such as sports drinks, cordials and soft drinks can also be used. They probably do not provide any physiological advantages in a non-endurance sport, but if you like the taste then you might be tempted to drink more—and look after your fluid needs better. Soft drinks and cordials are best diluted to half-strength to bring them into line with the sugar/glucose concentration that empties rapidly from your stomach.

### 4.7 Endurance events—fluid and food intakes

Events lasting over 90 minutes of continuous high-intensity exercise throw out a considerable challenge to competitors. Athletes in these sports will need a considered approach to fluid intake to keep pace with sweat losses. Depending on the pace of exercise, the environmental heat, and your size, over long-duration events, you can expect to sweat between 0.8 and 1.5 litres per hour. In most sports situations, a practical rule of thumb is to aim to replace about 80 per cent of sweat losses (as measured by body weight changes) as you go.

Many of these events will test the carbohydrate stores of the athlete, even when a full loading preparation has been undertaken. The best examples of this are long-distance running, ultradistance triathlons and long cycle races. Studies have shown that carbohydrate intake during this type of endurance event can improve performance. Once muscle glycogen stores have been depleted, a well-trained muscle can take up blood glucose at a sufficient rate to meet carbohydrate needs and continue exercise. A significant amount of carbohydrate is needed for this role—approximately 50g per hour, or about 1g per kilogram that you weigh. There is some evidence that in the most extreme conditions of prolonged intense exercise, when the depleted muscle is almost completely dependent on the bloodstream for its carbohydrate supply, that carbohydrate turnover can be higher still.

Carbohydrate intake during the event may also help to preserve blood glucose levels, preventing fatigue from hypoglycemia and ensuring that brain fuel is not in short supply. Since lowered blood glucose levels affect the brain and central nervous system, it is possible that reduced levels may interfere with skills and concentration, even before total fatigue becomes apparent. This may also be an advantage in team games and racquet sports that are played in lengthy sessions.

Theoretically, carbohydrate intake must start before the onset of fatigue, whether from depleted muscle glycogen stores or from lowered blood glucose levels. For some sports this might mean beginning carbohydrate intake in the middle or latter stages of the event, but other athletes may choose to take in carbohydrate at frequent intervals right from the start of exercise. In any case, once feeding has started it should continue to see out the event, and is better as a series of feeds rather than one giant load. How much carbohydrate you need to consume will depend on your muscles' fuel needs (how fast they are burning carbohydrate) and how well their own glycogen stores can meet this need. In less extreme sports you may find that 20–30g of carbohydrate per hour will be sufficient. However at the business end of a marathon or Ironman triathlon you may need every bit of a 50g per hour intake.

In various sports there are different traditions for taking in carbohydrate during events. For example, cyclists may eat Mars bars, sandwiches and bananas, while triathletes eat dried fruits, muesli bars and specially manufactured 'energy bars'. In cross-country skiing, thick sugary syrups are often drunk, while runners might try jelly beans—though more than a handful is required to supply 50g of carbohydrate.

In consuming carbohydrate during endurance exercise, an athlete must meet two conditions:

- the carbohydrate should not delay stomach emptying, thus interfering with fluid delivery as well;
- the carbohydrate should not cause gastrointestinal problems such as diarrhea from intestinal malabsorption or discomfort and nausea from stomach overfilling.

These issues will be most important in events that are carried out in hot weather—with greater fluid needs—and in events which involve high intensity exercise—with more likelihood of gastrointestinal discomfort. Gastrointestinal disturbances are more likely to occur in sports where the gut contents are joggled around, rather than sports that are played at low intensity or in a horizontal or gliding fashion. It is probably easier to swim or cycle with a couple of bananas in your stomach than to run a marathon! Of course, this is an individual characteristic of each athlete. Another factor recently identified as a cause of gastrointestinal disturbances is dehydration. This is especially interesting as some athletes do not take in fluids or food during exercise until they think they really need it—by which time they are already dehydrated. Many then attribute their stomach upset to the fluid they eventually drank, rather than to the fact that it was consumed too late.

Perhaps the most efficient and trouble-free way to provide carbohydrate and fluid needs simultaneously is by using sports drinks. In the past five years there has been much research to develop new products and to understand more about feeding athletes during exercise. Prior to this you might have been advised that sports drinks were too concentrated or too salty for use by athletes, and that if used they should be diluted.

We now know that well-trained athletes can empty quite a range of simple carbohydrate-based drinks from their stomachs—and of course any food or fluid must be emptied from the stomach before it can

## HINTS FOR INTAKE OF CARBOHYDRATE AND FLUID DURING ENDURANCE EVENTS

- Form a strategy to meet your expected fluid and fuel needs during the event. Look both to past experience in competition and to the arrangements that are proposed by event organisers.

- Practise in training with the types and amounts of fluids (or food) that you intend to use so that you can become an expert. Make sure that you enjoy the taste of your exercise refreshments.

- The theoretical nutritional requirements during endurance exercise are, per hour:

  - about 50g of carbohydrate
  - fluid intake to keep pace with sweat losses (aim to replace say 80 per cent of body weight losses). Under usual conditions, an intake of 500–800ml of fluid per hour will meet both fluid needs and a comfortable level of gastric filling and emptying. Under extreme conditions a gradual fluid deficit may still build up. Try to keep this under 2–3kg.

- Intake of fluid should begin early in the event and be taken at regular intervals as practical. An intake of 150–250ml of fluid every 15–20 minutes is a good benchmark.

- Cold fluids are more refreshing and palatable and may add an additional cooling effect.

- Don't let yourself become dehydrated. A reduced stomach-emptying rate plus an increased risk of gastrointestinal complaints will put you further behind in your exercise intake.

- The stomach empties fastest when it is fullest. In extremely hot conditions you may need to maximise fluid intake to meet extreme sweat losses. Make use of the 'volume effect' by starting the event with the largest amount of fluid in your stomach that can be comfortably tolerated. Top this up each 15–20 minutes as it empties, thus maximising gastric emptying rate and fluid intake.

- Carbohydrate intake may start simultaneously with fluid intake or may start later in the event. In any case, begin a significant intake before you start feeling fatigued, and continue throughout the event. Often, a sports drink consumed to meet fluid intake needs will also supply adequate carbohydrate intake.

- Although it is not necessary to use solid foods to provide carbohydrate requirements, many athletes will still enjoy the tradition or the convenience. If possible avoid carbohydrate foods that are high in fat and fibre, since these nutrients will delay gastric emptying. Experiment in training. Check the carbohydrate ready reckoner (Table 2.4) to find out how much food is needed to supply 50g of carbohydrate each hour.
- In events that last over 6–8 hours, it is possible that you will become 'hungry' and empty in the stomach. Where you are depending on carbohydrate drinks for fuel intake, a small amount of solid food can help to allay these feelings.
- A low level of electrolytes may be useful in an exercise fluid, especially during an ultra-endurance event. The sports drink is valuable for this reason.

become available to the rest of the body. Today's range of sports drinks generally fit the range of carbohydrate concentration (5–7 per cent solutions) that scientists have found to be well-tolerated. While some offer 'high-tech' ingredients such as glucose polymers which may have even greater advantages for stomach emptying, at the same time there are probably a dozen brands of sports drinks on the market that will meet the needs of athletes.

**Table 4.2  Analysis of some common sports drinks**

| Drink | | Carbohydrate | 50g CHO | Electrolytes |
|---|---|---|---|---|
| Bodyfuel | 7% | fructose glucose polymer | 700ml | sodium potassium |
| Exceed | 7% | glucose polymers fructose | 700ml | sodium potassium magnesium |
| Gatorade | 6% | sucrose glucose | 850ml | sodium potassium |
| Isostar | 6% | glucose polymer sucrose | 850ml | sodium potassium |
| Maximum | 7% | glucose polymers | 700ml | sodium potassium |
| Replace | 8% | glucose glucose polymers fructose | 650ml | sodium potassium magnesium |
| Staminade | 4% | glucose sucrose | 1250ml | sodium potassium |
| Suntory | 6.5% | sucrose glucose | 800ml | sodium potassium magnesium |

The characteristics of some sports drinks are summarised in Table 4.2. Note that an intake of 700–1000ml per hour of a sports drink will provide 50g of carbohydrate in addition to the fluid. An added extra, particularly for those in ultra-endurance events, is the addition of a small level of sodium and electrolytes. Although the optimal level of electrolytes has yet to be decided, sodium in an exercise drink may serve two useful purposes. First, it can increase intestinal absorption thus hastening fluid replacement and second, it may help to prevent the hyponatremia that occurs occasionally during ultra-endurance events. Providing you like the taste of the drink, a schedule of sports drinks can be a quick and easy way to take care of your exercise nutrition.

Generally, with shorter events, the duration prevents serious deficits of fluid or fuel from occuring. However, in endurance events, particularly those lasting over three hours at a high intensity, a definite plan of carbohydrate and fluid intake is required. It is not sufficient to drink or eat when you think you need it or when it is convenient. Form your strategy from the hints given.

# 5 Eating to recover

Being an athlete in the nineties means pushing yourself hard and long, striving to go beyond your best and hold it together until the finish. And then do it all over again tomorrow.

In many sports events, you may be required to compete more than once, with the interval between events being anything from 30 minutes to 24 hours. For example, you may be racing in an athletics carnival where you have to run in heats, semi-finals and even the final in the one day. In a basketball or tennis tournament you may be scheduled for one or two games each day. A cycle tour may be composed of one or two stages each day, lasting for a week or more. Indeed, the training schedules of many athletes pose a similar challenge to optimise recovery between sessions, particularly when two or even three hard sessions are planned each day. In all cases, performance is dependent on your ability to recover from one session and present yourself at your best for the next.

In the nineties, recovery should be regarded as an active part of training or competition. It is no longer passive, happening by itself, in its own good time. Rather, special strategies are employed to speed up recovery processes and promote the level of return. There are many components to this, including massage, relaxation and sleep. Nutritional recovery includes:

- replacing the fluid and electrolytes lost in sweat
- refuelling muscle glycogen stores
- repairing any damage caused by the exercise and building new structures to adapt to the workload.

The peak training diet includes active recovery in its checklist of goals. In the main, your eating patterns should now provide all the building blocks and the vitamins and minerals necessary to build and repair. These processes probably happen over a longer time frame than the acute challenges of rehydrating and refuelling. Recent scientific studies have focused on the acute situation to find special strategies to enhance these recovery issues—not just what to eat and drink, but when to do it!

## 5.1 Restoring fluid and electrolyte balance

Even where planned fluid intake has been carried out before and during an exercise session—either competition or training—it is likely that you will still finish the session with some degree of dehydration. This is particularly true for prolonged and intense sessions in a hot environment, where sweat losses exceed the usual intake of fluid. However, this may also be expected in short events where there is little or no opportunity for fluid intake during exercise. If you are required to compete or train again within a short period, whether hours later or the next day, it is important that fluid levels be restored.

Most athletes will not be fully aware of the degree of dehydration that has occurred during a session. Human beings have a poor in-built ability to gauge and repair this, so it is better to rely on an objective assessment and a definite plan of attack, rather than simply listening to thirst. The amount of fluid needed to restore fluid levels may vary from 500ml to three litres, depending on how much sweat you lost during the session, and how well you attempted to replace it during the exercise itself. A quick guide to dehydration state is to weigh yourself before and after the session—minus sweaty clothes, of course. A kilogram of lost weight is roughly equal to a litre of fluid that needs to be replaced—except in endurance events where you weighed in heavier than normal with loaded glycogen stores. If you carbo-loaded before the event, subtract 1–2kg from your pre-event weight to account for the extra glycogen, leaving you with true fluid losses. Alternatively, go by your usual training weight.

Any fluid, taken in sufficient quantities, will contribute significantly towards restoring fluid balance after exercise. Water is probably the most accessible and practical rehydrater for most situations. However, there is some evidence that a sports drink, containing moderate amounts of carbohydrate and a small level of electrolytes will actually speed up the restoration of fluid balance when a large deficit has been created. Sodium in the fluid may help to increase the rate of intestinal uptake of fluid, and also increase the rate at which blood volume returns to normal levels.

This would be useful in situations where the athlete is significantly dehydrated (say, where fluid deficit is more than three litres) or where rapid hydration is required before the next event. A good example is a tennis tournament where matches are played out for many hours on a hot court, and the winner must go on to play again. Also, in such severely challenging situations quick carbohydrate replacement will probably also be of benefit, so a sports drink can fulfil a number of roles. The electrolytes may go towards the general replacement of salts lost during the exercise, but their most important role is probably to aid the restoration of fluid balance.

The best time to start drinking is straight away, and you may need to continue your drinking plan throughout the day to replace large fluid deficits. Some organisation may be needed to have the fluids cold, refreshing and available. Plan ahead for your post-exercise requirements—you may need to bring some drinks down to the session—and for the rest of the day if necessary. A jug on your desk at work, or at the front of the fridge can help to remind you of the task in hand.

Lastly, don't forget that other post-exercise practices may work against your hydration plans. Staying in a hot environment will continue to make you sweat. Avoid sitting in the sun to watch how other competitors are faring or spending long hours in the hot tub or spa. Alcohol and caffeine-containing beverages will act as a diuretic rather than a fluid replacer, so be wary drinking these in large quantities.

## 5.2 Replacing glycogen stores

Depending on the length and intensity of the training session or competition event, it is likely that your muscle glycogen stores will need a top-up before the next exercise session. This calls for strategies to maximise glycogen synthesis. The amount of dietary carbohydrate needed to secure maximum daily glycogen storage was given in Chapter 2—an estimated 9–10g per kilogram you weigh each day.

Figure 5.1 shows the now classic illustration of daily muscle glycogen replacement, comparing the carbohydrate intake of the typical Australian diet (40–45 per cent of energy), with the high-carbohydrate recommendations. Athletes with a prolonged and intense daily exercise schedule, whether in training or in the competition setting, should aim for these targets. Failure to meet these daily intakes may impede recovery and prevent good performance on subsequent days. The effect can be quite dramatic or gradual, perhaps invisible—but nevertheless, the Wall.

It is not just the total amount of carbohydrate eaten after exhaustive exercise that determines muscle glycogen recovery. A recent study has shown that timing of carbohydrate intake is a crucial factor in the recovery process. Researchers found that when carbohydrate was eaten immediately after exhaustive exercise, there was immediate and rapid synthesis of muscle glycogen—twice as fast as when carbohydrate intake was delayed until two hours after the session (Figure 5.2).

This makes sense when you consider that your muscles will remain active for a short time after the exercise has finished—blood flow will continue to be diverted to the muscles and the muscle cells will continue to welcome glucose uptake across their membranes. After about two hours, it seems that this window of opportunity is closed and the muscle returns to a lower level of activity. To take advantage of the higher activity state, you must deliver some carbohydrate building blocks to the muscle as soon as the exercise session has finished.

Of course, in real life this crucial time is usually when the athlete

**Figure 5.1 Daily recovery from prolonged exercise**

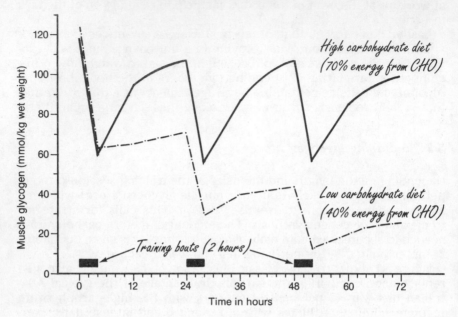

*Prolonged daily exercise sessions gradually lead to low glycogen levels when the typical Australian diet (low carbohydrate) is eaten. Switching to a high carbohydrate diet helps to promote daily recovery of muscle glycogen stores.*

Source: D. L. Costill and J. M. Miller, *International Journal of Sports Medicine*, 12–14, 1980

has least opportunity or desire to eat. You may not have access to food (or the right food) at the track, the field, or the velodrome. You may be tied up with post-competition officialdom, or have a tight schedule of stretching, cleaning your equipment and driving to your next commitment after training. Perhaps you feel nauseous, or too tired to eat, let alone prepare a meal.

Again, good planning comes into play. Bringing your own food and drink to the competition site can be a good move. You can munch away while you attend to your other commitments. Simple and easy-to-eat foods may be the order of the day, especially when you are feeling exhausted.

How much carbohydrate is needed to get an effect? Studies suggest that you should eat about 1g of carbohydrate per kg of body weight within the first 10–15 minutes after exercise, and again every two hours until you get back into your normal high carbohydrate meal

**Figure 5.2 Short-term recovery after prolonged exercise**

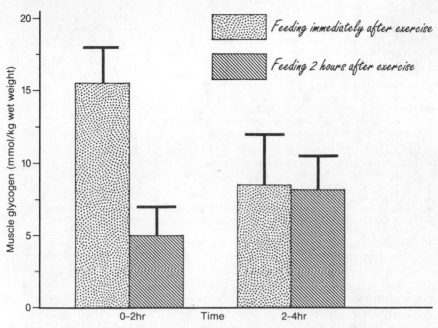

*You can speed up the recovery of muscle glycogen stores after prolonged exercise, by eating carbohydrate foods immediately after you finish.*
*Waiting for a couple of hours before you eat will mean a slower recovery rate.*

Source: J. Ivy et al, *Journal of Applied Physiology*, 64 : 1480–5, 1988

routine. This will mean 50–100g of carbohydrate at each snack depending on your size. Table 5.1 lists some 50g carbohydrate snacks to help you achieve this target. Investigations are being carried out to see whether certain carbohydrate foods promote faster glycogen synthesis than others. However, until this is known, choose your carbohydrate snacks according to the following rules-of-thumb:

• For acute or one-off situations where replacing muscle glycogen is the absolute priority, choose the most practical and easy to eat carbohydrate choices.

• If this carbohydrate intake is contributing significantly to your overall diet (i.e. if you are a low energy consumer, or you need to practise glycogen storing strategies day in, day out) then you should choose the more nutritious carbohydrate choices.

**Table 5.1   Examples of 50g carbohydrate snacks**

Light and easy to eat:
- 250ml of carbo-loader supplement (Gatorlode, Exceed High Carbohydrate source)
- 250–350ml of liquid meal supplement (Exceed Sports Nutrition Supplement or Sustagen) or a home-made low-fat milk shake/fruit smoothie
- 800–1000ml of sports drink
- 800ml of cordial
- 500ml of fruit juice, soft drink or flavoured mineral water
- 50g packet of jelly beans or jelly lollies
- 1 round of jam sandwiches (thick-sliced bread and lots of jam!)
- 3 medium pieces of fruit (e.g. apple, orange and banana)
- Large Mars Bar (70g)—note that this is a high-fat choice
- 3 Muesli bars—also high in fat if choc-coated

Quick, low-fat and nutritious:
- 250–350ml of liquid meal supplement (Exceed Sports Nutrition Supplement or Sustagen) or a home-made low-fat milk shake/fruit smoothie
- Cup of thick vegetable soup with a wholemeal roll
- Salad sandwich and a piece of fruit
- Carton of low fat fruit yoghurt and a muesli bar (not chocolate)
- Large baked potato (250–300g) with low-fat filling and a glass of skim milk
- Bowl of cereal with skim milk
- Bowl of fruit salad with 1/2 carton of low-fat fruit yoghurt

For example, immediately after the event you may choose an easy-to-eat carbohydrate snack, not worrying about its total nutritional value. The most obvious choice is, of course, a carbohydrate drink, which looks after fluid and carbohydrate needs simultaneously. After this you might then get back into the nutritious carbohydrate choices, which are already the mainstay of your peak training diet.

A final word about muscle glycogen recovery. Muscle damage—either through eccentric exercise or through direct body contact and bruising—will delay muscle glycogen synthesis. Studies have shown that the amount and timing of carbohydrate intake is even more crucial for damaged muscles. Muscle glycogen recovery seems most affected after 24 hours—the time that you are probably experiencing the delayed muscle soreness that follows eccentric exercise such as hard running or some weight training exercises. The message is to pay special attention to a high post-exercise carbohydrate intake, especially over the first 24 hours when the muscles will respond more efficiently.

### 5.3   Multi-event competitions

There are a great variety of competition situations and schedules that require an athlete to compete over and over. Between events you will need to consider recovery from the first session, and then specific preparation for the second. In some ways, good recovery leaves you well-prepared. The fine-tuning is to add the pre-event meal strategies

**Table 5.2  Nutritional practices for various competition schedules**

| Description | Strategies |
|---|---|
| Short intense events repeated in the same day (swimming meet, weightlifting competition, etc) | Replace mild to moderate fluid losses between events, and top up body carbohydrate stores over the day with a schedule of carbohydrate drinks or foods. Drinks will be handy when there is only a short interval between events, and where solid food may lead to gut discomfort. When you have more time between events (e.g. heats and finals) a carbohydrate snack or meal may be suitable. Liquid meal supplements (e.g. Sustagen, Exceed Sports Nutrition Supplements) can provide a half-way point, being more substantial than other drinks, but less upsetting than solids. Take extra care if you have dehydrated slightly to meet a weigh-in target, and be prepared to bring your own food and fluid supplies to the competition. Not all venues will cater adequately for your nutritional needs. |
| Moderate length events repeated in the same day (e.g. badminton or basketball 'lightning' championship) | The same principles apply as above, but you may need to work harder to replace both fluid and carbohydrate stores. Make sure that you start your plan straight after the event. |
| Moderate length events over successive days (e.g. basketball or waterpolo tournament) | During the day you may follow the same schedule as above. Once competition is over for the day you can turn your attention to preparing for the next day. Again, plan a post-event carbohydrate top-up, and make sure that all sweat losses are replaced. Meal schedules may need to be flexible if your events are held at different times each day. Pay attention to including nutritious food choices as well as using convenient carbohydrate and fluid forms. |
| Prolonged events over successive days (e.g. cycle tour, tennis tournament) | It will be a challenge to meet fluid and fuel needs both during events and between events. Sports supplements may be useful in many situations—e.g. carbohydrate drinks during competition, and low bulk 'carbo-loader' and liquid meal supplements as a boost to food intake when the day is over. |

covered in Chapter 4. Your overall strategies will vary according to the following features:

• The physiological requirements of the event—the length, intensity and type of exercise will decide both the level and type of depletion or fatigue that must be recovered from the initial event, as well as the limiting factors that must be prevented or postponed in the next event.

• The interval between events—this will decide how much recovery time you have, and whether you need to juggle solid food and drinks to avoid gut discomfort.

- The signficance of total nutritional goals—if an athlete competes periodically in events over a couple of days, then it may be sufficient to concentrate on immediate fluid and carbohydrate issues. However, if competition extends over weeks, or makes up a significant proportion of the athlete's training life, then total nutritional goals, such as vitamin, protein and mineral needs, will have to be taken into account.

Look at your competition schedule to plot out the times of your events and the intervals in between. Table 5.2 lists some common event time-tables and the typical nutrition issues that arise. Juggling these issues is often a challenging business. There is probably no single perfect system, but there are two overriding rules:

1 Experiment until you find the system that works for you and your sport. Practise in training to be sure.

2 Be prepared to organise your own supplies to make it happen on the day. Don't leave anything to chance or to the event organisers. Be in control.

# 6   Pills and potions

It is hard to open a sports magazine without being bombarded with advertisements for nutritional supplements—all promising to make you bigger, stronger, leaner, faster or whatever it takes to be a better athlete in your sport. How can you refuse such a tempting offer? Or, better still, how can you afford to let your competitor get an edge that you don't have?

In 1983, a survey of over 4000 Australian athletes reported that 47 per cent were regular users of nutritional supplements. Each year billions of dollars are spent in search of a bottle of the 'Winning Edge', and each decade a new set of wonder substances replaces the last set. Do they work? That is the question of the nineties.

## 6.1   Why do athletes use supplements?

There are three basic reasons why athletes turn to supplements and these need to be considered separately:

1   They consider that they eat poorly or perhaps they have an in-adequate lifestyle. Wrong! How can some extra vitamins make up for late nights, too much alcohol or too much fat in your diet? There is only one solution to these problems—face the real issue and fix up your act properly!

2   They consider that their nutritional requirements for sport are too great, or their food supply is too low in nutritional value to meet their needs. Occasionally perhaps. But has a dietitian helped you to make best use of the food supply before you turn to supple-ments? And have you been advised about the right supplement for any remaining shortcomings?

3   They consider that some supplements can directly enhance sport performance. Maybe. But when, which ones and how much?

To sort out the answers, it helps to divide the large variety of supple-ments on the market into two categories: dietary supplements and nutritional ergogenic aids.

## 6.2   Dietary supplements in sport

A dietary supplement can be described by the following features:

• most commonly, it contains nutrients in amounts similar to the Recommended Dietary Intakes (RDIs) and to the amounts found in

**Table 6.1  Some dietary supplements and their uses in sport**

| Supplement | Uses |
|---|---|
| Sports drinks (carbohydrate–electrolyte drinks) | • Endurance exercise—fluid and carbohydrate replacement<br>• Post-exercise recovery—rehydration and glycogen resynthesis |
| Liquid meal supplements (e.g. Sustagen, Exceed Sports Nutrition Supplement) | • Training diet—support high-energy, high-nutrient needs<br>• Competition preparation—low-residue meal for empty gut<br>• Pre-competition meal |
| High carbohydrate supplements (e.g. Gatorlode, Exceed High Carbohydrate Source) | • Carbohydrate loading<br>• Post-exercise recovery—glycogen resynthesis |
| Multivitamin/mineral supplement (low dose, broad range) | • Supplement dietary intake to meet nutrient RDIs |
| Iron supplement | • High dose—treat iron deficiency<br>• Low dose—supplement dietary intake to meet iron requirements |
| Calcium supplement | • Supplement diet to meet calcium requirements and promote calcium balance |

food, and provides these nutrients in a form that is practical or convenient for a sports situation;

• alternatively, it contains large amounts of a nutrient, specifically for the rapid treatment of a nutritional deficiency;

• rather than being 'magic', it is seen as being a means to an end, by being used to respond to a nutritional need or challenge that arises in sport—and by doing so, help the athlete to achieve peak performance;

• it is supported by scientific trials and studies, and has the interest and approval of mainstream science.

Examples of dietary supplements are found in Table 6.1, with the situations in which they may contribute to sports performance. Some can be used to directly enhance exercise performance—for example, the sports drink—while others are used to contribute to the athlete's overall nutritional status and, therefore, indirectly contribute to peak performance.

Note that in all cases it is not the supplement that 'works', but rather the success of the athlete in understanding their nutritional goals and matching the supplement to the situation. The right supplement must be used at the right place at the right time, and in the right amounts. For example, an iron supplement will only benefit an athlete who is truly iron deficient, and can only reverse the deficiency when used in the correct dose for an appropriate time. A sports drink will not improve performance in a 100m sprint event, where the nutritional requirements for fluid and carbohydrate replacement have not been created. Some of these supplements and their application to particular sports will be discussed in Part II of this book. Talk to a sports dietitian if you are not sure how to make best use of these supplements in your situation.

Dietary supplements deal with well-known and well-studied nutritional and physiological challenges in sport. Scientific trials are continually being conducted to develop and support supplements and their strategies of use. Many of the supplements are produced by large pharmaceutical companies who contribute towards the research and provide nutrition education for athletes. This shows a good balance between the needs of the company, the athlete and the exercise scientist.

## 6.3 *Nutritional ergogenic aids*

By definition, an ergogenic aid is something that directly improves work output, or exercise performance. A nutritional ergogenic aid is a supplement containing a nutrient or food-related substance, eaten in the hope of an immediate boost to performance. It is these supplements that have captured the imagination (and wallets) of the athletic world. A general description includes many of the following features:

- it contains nutrients or other substances in much larger quantities than the RDIs or the amounts normally found in food;
- it aims to produce a pharmacological or (legal) drug-like action to improve performance. In other words, the action is outside the known physiological role of the substance;
- it is backed by a proposed mechanism that may sound scientific but is often untested. Where trials have been undertaken, most fail to detect an ergogenic effect. In fact by strict definition, 'proposed ergogenic aid' might be a better title for many supplements, since there is no certainty of their effectiveness.
- it is generally not supported by mainstream science;
- it is often manufactured by small companies who have no pharmaceutical expertise and who fail to support research;
- it comes and goes in fashion;
- it can be expensive.

A quick guide to some currently popular nutritional ergogenic aids, and the available scientific evidence, is presented in Table 6.2. The question of cost is covered in Figure 6.1 which examines the cost of a popular supplement against a similar amount from a food source. If

**Table 6.2  Some popular nutritional ergogenic aids**

| | |
|---|---|
| Vitamins—megadoses | The most popular and enduring of the ergogenic aids. The role of vitamins at RDI levels has been well established. Following the 'if a little is good, more is better' rule, almost all of the vitamins have been tried in large doses, in the hope of an extra boost to performance. Vitamins C, E and the B group have been studied in scientific trials. To date, the evidence fails to support an ergogenic effect. |
| Protein powders | Promoted to boost muscle mass. In Chapter 3, the principles of muscle gain were outlined: the right genetic potential, a strength training program, and a high-energy, high-nutrient diet. If you need a supplement to boost dietary intake, go for a complete nutrition aid (liquid meal supplements) rather than the more expensive protein-only supplements. |
| Amino acids | Amino acids are the building blocks of protein. However, amino acid supplements are not intended as a general protein supplement. Instead, the various preparations contain individual amino acids (singly or in groups), each suggested to have a special 'mission'. For example, arginine and ornithine are suggested to promote growth hormone release, thus 'legally' stimulating muscle growth. The branched-chain amino acids are proposed to enhance recovery. While amino acids are currently the hottest property on the supplement scene, scientific studies have yet to validate the testimonials from some athletes. |
| Caffeine | Caffeine occurs naturally in coffee, tea and cola drinks, and may also be found in over-the-counter pharmaceutical preparations. The main interest in caffeine and exercise lies in the endurance arena. Studies have shown, particularly with cycling, that caffeine taken an hour before prolonged exercise increases the time to fatigue. One theory is that caffeine stimulates fat metabolism during endurance exercise, sparing muscle glycogen stores. However, other studies show different results. Like most drugs, caffeine elicits a variety of responses in people, and whether caffeine improves your exercise performance—even to perk up your central nervous system to make you feel less tired—may be individual to you. Experiment for yourself. However, be wary of possible side-effects—caffeine is a diuretic and may add to your dehydration problems. And caffeine is no longer a legal drug in sport. A urinary concentration of over 12 micrograms per ml is deemed a positive test for caffeine doping. Your usual morning cup poses no threat, however—you would need to consume 6–8 cups of coffee or 10 cans of cola in a short time to reach this level. |
| Bicarbonate | Sports lasting for 2–5 minutes of intense exercise are usually affected by the build-up of lactic acid. Remember the burning feeling? By adding more buffer to the blood to mop up the acidity, it is thought that fatigue might be delayed. Some studies have shown that bicarbonate taken before events such as an 800m run, a rowing race, or a 400m swim, does the job and improves performance. However, like caffeine, there seems to be a narrow range of conditions and individuals who benefit. Side effects include gut discomfort and diarrhea. You will have to practise bicarbonate loading yourself to decide if it helps your performance (of course, try it in training first). |

**Table 6.2 (Continued)**

| | |
|---|---|
| Bee pollen | Bee pollen offers a glamourous and exotic approach to performance enhancement. However, there is doubt over the real composition of some supplements. This might explain why the controlled trials have failed to find any improvement after taking bee pollen. |
| Carnitine | Carnitine is a carrier molecule which transports fat into the cell's energy chambers to be metabolised. Your body manufactures its own supply. A popular theory of weight-losers is that extra carnitine might speed up the delivery of fat, and the fat-burning process itself. It might also help the endurance athlete to burn more fat during prolonged exercise, again saving precious glycogen. Too good to be true? The studies that have been conducted show conflicting results. It seems too early to make a decision about the value of carnitine. |
| Coenzyme Q10, ATP | ATP is the final product in the cell's metabolic pathway to energy. Wouldn't it be good if you could jump the queue and get straight to the business end of energy production! There are a number of 'metabolic enhancer' products containing ATP or substances such as Coenzyme Q10 which are involved in the last steps of energy liberation. To date there is little evidence to support any ergogenic effect. |
| Inosine | Inosine is another proclaimed energy enhancer, because of its links with ATP production and the red blood cell lifecycle. Studies have not been able to transform this theory into a substantiated performance-enhancing practice. In addition, there are some questions about the safety of inosine, because of possible connections with gout. |
| Ginseng | There is a long list of wonders attributed to this herb, and a number of 'active ingredients' have been identified. However, studies have generally failed to detect any performance changes in athletes using ginseng. Problems with standardising the composition of supplements makes the study process difficult. |
| 'Vitamin' B15 | Despite the well-known name, this substance is not a real vitamin. It has not proved successful in scientific trials with athletes. |

you buy these supplements, do ever ask yourself who is pocketing the cash?

Because there is no regulation of the nutritional supplement industry, at least at present, there is no legal requirement for a company to provide proof of its claims. Until the law—or the athlete—demands proof, there will be no clear answer to the question 'does it work?' To be fair, we still don't know that ergogenic aids do *not* work, but nor do we know if they are harmful or have side-effects. In an ideal world, supplement manufacturers would co-operate with scientists and athletes to carefully study the supplements and hunt for the answers.

What, then, is the basis of proof?

**Figure 6.1  Cost of supplements vs. nutrients from food**

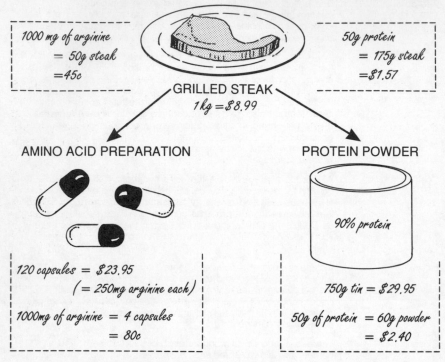

1000 mg of arginine
= 50g steak
=45c

50g protein
= 175g steak
=$1.57

GRILLED STEAK
1kg =$8.99

AMINO ACID PREPARATION

PROTEIN POWDER

90% protein

120 capsules = $23.95
( = 250mg arginine each)
1000mg of arginine = 4 capsules
= 80c

750g tin = $29.95

50g of protein = 60g powder
= $2.40

*A 50g serve of protein provided by a popular protein powder, is more expensive than an equivalent protein serve from lean steak.*

*A typically recommended dose of the amino acid, arginine, can be found at less cost in a 50g serve of meat.*

*Not only is the food source cheaper, but think of all the other nutrients you get at the same time.*

### 6.4  How do you prove something works?

*The scientific theory*

The mode of action of an ergogenic aid must be explainable—there must be some sort of scientific rationale to support how or why the supplement works. In the case of the dietary supplements this is easier, since they operate in the realms of exercise physiology that we already understand. However, many of the nutritional ergogenic aids are based on quite complicated manipulations of biochemical reactions. Many of the substances are found as coenzymes, cofactors and other products of the metabolic pathways of exercise. The basis of many of these 'scientific theories' is that if you provide much larger doses of some compounds to the cells, metabolism will proceed faster and longer, thus improving performance. Sounds good on paper doesn't it?

Therein lies the problem. A little science can be a dangerous thing when it is extrapolated by someone who can't look at all sides of the situation properly. The full scientific perspective may require the input of a range of specialists trained in human physiology and digestion, exercise physiology, enzyme kinetics and biochemistry. The human body is a complex unit, and many steps occur between popping a tablet into your mouth and having something happen in your muscle cells. Even if a substance might enhance metabolism from *inside* the cell, the experts may tell you that this substance won't be able to pass through your digestive system intact, or that the molecule is too big to pass across the cell membrane to get inside. In other words, eating large amounts of the substance is not necessarily going to work as you first thought.

A theory is just that—a theory. It is the first line of enquiry, but should never stand alone as proof. When experts have judged it from all angles, and found it to hold some possibilities, then the next stage is to put it under the scrutiny of the scientific trial.

### Personal endorsements and anecdotal stories

In the eyes of the athlete, the most powerful proof that a supplement works is the endorsement of another athlete—particularly an elite athlete. If your hero swears that 'Product X' helped him to win the world championship, you will at least be interested, if not sold on the the supplement. If you don't believe how emotive this is, just look at how the ergogenic aid companies advertise.

Not all the personal endorsements for ergogenic aids are paid for or appear in glossy full-page ads. Athletes are continually searching for the winning edge, and many conduct their own supplement trials— with a study population of one! The results are rapidly spread by word-of-mouth. How does this stand up as proof? What does it mean if you, or the world's greatest swimmer, or the school's football team performed well while taking 'Product X'? Unfortunately, under the scientific microscope it means little. It is equally possible that you would have performed as well without Product X, or in some cases even in spite of it.

For a start, performance is multifactorial. It is affected by your equipment, your diet, training methods, natural ability, mental attitude, sleep, and the environment. It is almost impossible in real life to control all these factors so that the effect of the supplement can be judged on its own. You might have ridden a faster time in the triathlon this year, but how much of this is due to Product X, and how much is due to the extra year of training, your new aerodynamic handle bars, and the tail wind?

Secondly, there is the placebo effect. This describes the ability of your mind, when you really believe in something, to make it come true—even for a short period of time. It has been well-documented that when a group of people are given a tablet, and sold on the story of how it will work, a large number of that group will report that the effect actually happened, even when the tablet only contains sugar. Sometimes they can create the effect themselves, sometimes they just believe that it has occurred. Just like a rabbit's foot, or your 'lucky underwear', a supplement can provoke a psychologically-powered improvement even without a physiologically-based reason.

So personal experiences can create the next level of interest in an ergogenic aid—but however impressive they sound, there is no real seal of approval until scientific trials have been done.

## The scientific trial

A well-conducted scientific trial remains our best hope of substantiating the claims about supplements—whether dietary supplements or the ergogenic-aid type. However, such trials must be carried out with extreme care and strict guidelines. They should involve a large number of subjects, and be designed to mimic a real sports situation with relevant physiological and performance changes.

A dummy supplement should be used in a scientific trial to counter the placebo effect. The subjects should be divided into two groups with one receiving the real supplement and the other the dummy. Neither the subjects nor the testers should know which is which until the end—in this way no-one can bias the experiment and its results.

Sometimes the trial is conducted twice in each group, switching the tablets over so that each group has one period on the real substance and one on the dummy. With this cross-over, each subject acts as their own comparison or control, thus cancelling out some of the individual factors that effect performance. In all scientific studies, much effort should be aimed at controlling other performance variables. Lastly, for a fair trial, the scientist should be sure to test the supplement in a dose, a duration, and with the type of subjects in which changes are most likely to occur.

These criteria obviously mean that a good study is time consuming, expensive to run and requires a great deal of co-operation from subjects. It is not hard to see why so few studies have been done, or why questions are not fully answered when a study has a few flaws. Until the ideal world is created—with scientists, athletes and supplement companies joining force to provide the scientific answers—the decision about using nutritional ergogenic aids rests with you.

## 6.5  *Making your own decision about ergogenic aids*

The positive side about the large array of nutritional ergogenic aids is the chance that one or more, might actually improve your performance, whether by real action or by the placebo effect.

What are the costs of being a human guinea pig? Firstly, there may be side-effects from the long-term and heavy use of some products. If they are as powerful as they are reported to be, then how do you know that all the effects will be in your favour? All nutritional ergogenic aids, including vitamins, are chemicals—too much of any chemical can cause problems. Ergogenic aids will certainly effect your wallet, as many are extremely expensive and many athletes use a number of products.

By strict definition, an ergogenic aid causes a pharmacological or a 'legal drug' effect. There is always the possibility that any substances that are found to directly improve performance will then be judged as unfair in competition and subsequently banned. Already, many sports bodies have deemed that large doses of caffeine constitute 'doping'.

Finally, don't pin your hopes on the ergogenic aid and overlook factors that definitely affect performance. There is no pill or potion that can replace good training, an optimal training diet, a strong mental attitude, and adequate sleep and recovery.

# II  Sports nutrition in action

# Introduction

In this section we will turn theory into practice, by looking inside a number of sports to see the nutritional challenges faced by athletes. Typical nutrition issues arising from the physiological requirements of training and competition as well as the lifestyle of the athlete will be identified.

These sports were chosen to represent a variety of different nutrition issues. If your sport has not been specifically covered, you will probably find that you can identify with another sport, or with various issues that arise in a combination of sports. Think about the features of your sport—both the characteristics of competition and the way that you train. By reading the brief description at the beginning of each chapter you may be able to identify another sport (or group of sports) that makes similar demands as your field. Alternatively, you may already know some of the nutrition issues that interest and concern you. Use the index at the back of the book to find where these are covered—particularly in the form of a case history. For example, loss of body fat is a goal shared by athletes in many sports, and even if you are a lacrosse player you may be able to identify with the weight loss efforts of Vicki the netballer. Similarly, if you are vegetarian or thinking of becoming one, you will find Maureen's experiences of interest in the gymnastics chapter, and the hints for the travelling athlete in the tennis chapter will be valuable no matter what your sport is.

Finally, appreciate that each chapter covers *typical* issues, and is by no means complete or exclusive. Your nutrition goals and interests may be a little different to those in the chapter on your sport. Hopefully, however, you will find something that addresses you personally and individually. Above all, enjoy this section for the chance to think about the practical and human aspects of nutrition for sport. It should help you to convert science into food choices and eating habits, and thus help you to take your sport as far as your ambitions reach.

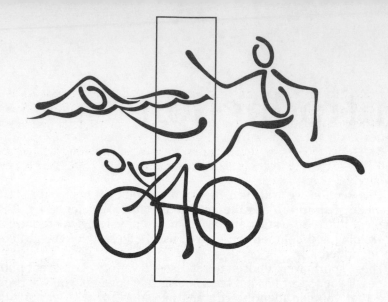

# Triathlon

Triathlon has been described as the boom sport of the 1980s. In this multi-sport event, competitors complete a swim, cycle and run in immediate succession, with races broadly categorised as follows:

Short course: 500m swim/20km cycle/5km run
Olympic distance: 1.5km swim/40km cycle/10km run
Long course: 2km swim/80km cycle/20km run
Ultra distance/Ironman: 3.9km swim/180km cycle/42.2km run.

At present men dominate the race numbers, with women making up 10–15 per cent of the field. In most triathlons, all competitors race alongside each other, with a prize structure that recognises males and females, elite and recreational, as well as different age groups. There are not too many sports that allow everyday athletes to toe the starting line with their heroes!

### Training

It is not surprising with three sports to master that triathlon training can be time-consuming. Even recreational triathletes can spend more that ten hours each week in training, and top competitors may spend 20–40 hours—a full-time job! Typical weekly totals for a serious Olympic-distance triathlete are 10km swimming, 200km cycling and 40km running. A triathlete specialising in longer events may more than double this load.

The bulk of triathlon training is aerobic, with interval training being included in some sessions. Many triathletes include transition training in their schedules, with one sport being immediately followed by another (usually a cycle followed by a run). Weight training is sometimes included when time and facilities permit.

The most important fuel for training is muscle glycogen, and intense daily training will challenge the recovery of stores in the various muscle groups involved in each sport.

## Competition

The official triathlon season extends from late spring to early autumn. Events are held on weekends (usually Sundays) and are held early in the morning to avoid the heat. During winter, when open water swims are impractical, triathletes may compete in run-ride-run races (duathlons). Elite triathletes may compete internationally in an almost year-round circuit.

Triathletes vary with their competition schedules. Some triathletes specialise in a set distance (either short or long course) while others compete over all race distances. Some athletes compete most weekends during competition season, up to 20 times a year, but select a handful of key races to taper for. Others choose to spread their races over the season. Juggling competition and training schedules can present a great challenge to many athletes.

Triathlons are predominantly an aerobic event, with short course races taking as little as 45 minutes to complete, while ultra distance events take eight hours at best—and considerably longer for most competitors. A triathlon can be conducted at a higher intensity than a single sport of the same time duration and is less likely to be limited by the depletion of fuel stores, since the work is spread over a larger number of muscle groups. However, in longer triathlons the individual distances in each sport will challenge the fuel stores in the muscles involved, as well as the body's ability to maintain blood glucose levels.

The duration and environment of triathlons are important factors in terms of fluid loss and temperature regulation. While some triathlons threaten competitors with possible cold exposure and hypothermia, in most triathlons the problem of dehydration and heat distress are a greater risk. The famous Ironman race held in Hawaii each year challenges athletes not only with the long distances, but with strong winds and ground temperatures of over 40 degrees Celsius.

## Physical characteristics

The only spare tyres that elite triathletes carry are under their bike saddles in case of a puncture! Like distance running, triathlon performance is advantaged by a low level of body fat, so elite triathletes have similarly low skinfold levels to elite marathon runners. However, because swimming makes active use of upper body muscle mass, the total muscle mass and body weight of a triathlete will be greater than that of the marathon runner, with the greater muscle mass being found around the chest, arms and shoulders.

## Common nutrition issues

### Dietary extremism

Triathletes are renowned for their enthusiasm and self-discipline. They don't do things by half measures, and that includes diet. Many triathletes read widely about nutrition, including alternative diets such as vegetarianism and Pritikin. Some become skilled headhunters of 'bad foods' which are then single-mindedly eliminated from their diets. The result of this excessiveness is a restricted dietary range, causing a number of problems and missed opportunities (see the account of Victor at the end of this chapter). The most important rule of the peak training diet is to enjoy a variety of foods. Read Chapter 1 to see how this can be achieved while meeting all other nutritional goals for training.

### Excessively low body-fat levels

Also along the lines of 'too much of a good thing', a current fashion in triathlon is to strive for the lowest level of body fat possible. This sometimes happens as a consequence of dietary extremism, but is often pursued as a goal in itself.

Triathletes should recognise firstly that optimum body-fat levels are individual, and that it is not necessarily an advantage to have the body-fat levels of Mark Allen or Dave Scott—unless you are Mark Allen or Dave Scott. Secondly, for *all* triathletes, optimum body-fat level includes the issue of good health. If your body fat drops to a level that causes problems with cold intolerance, loss of immune function and loss of strength/muscle mass, then this is *not* your optimum body-fat level—even if it does mean less 'dead weight' to carry over the course (see Chapter 3.1).

### High energy requirements

The intense training program of a triathlete, especially the full-time or elite athlete, will chalk up massive energy requirements. This is how most triathletes natually achieve their low body-fat levels. However, sometimes when a triathlete begins a training program, or increases the training load, body weight can drop below a desirable level. There are a number of reasons why food intake does not automatically adjust itself to meet the increased requirements of training. Being too extreme with food range has already been nominated; other factors include being too tired after training to cook, or even to eat. The bulk of the high-carbohydrate, high-fibre diet is often self limiting, especially when the athlete has to juggle eating times around work and training schedules (see Chapter 3.7 for smart ways to increase energy intake by eating 'compact' kilojoules and by increasing the number of meals rather than their size).

### Loss of body fat

Sometimes, despite heavy training, a triathlete will need additional help to reduce body-fat levels. For some, this is a constant struggle. Females in particular, seem to need to eat less kilojoules than their training loads would predict. If you are a lower-than-expected energy consumer, you may find it frustrating when fellow athletes eat twice as much as you, or enjoy the feeding frenzies otherwise known as carbo-loading banquets, without gaining a gram. Chapter 3.3 will show you how to concentrate your efforts on a weight loss program and an energy intake level that is suitable for you.

### Iron status

Triathletes, especially females, are in the high risk group for iron deficiency problems. The early stages of iron deficiency may reduce the ability to recover between training sessions, even before full-blown anemia causes a definite reduction in exercise performance. As discussed in Chapter 2.5, hard-training triathletes may experience increased iron requirements, perhaps due to increased iron losses from gut bleeding and red blood cell loss. However, the factor most likely to contribute to iron deficiency problems is the low intake of well-absorbed iron in the typical triathlete's diet. Read Chapter 2.5 to make sure that you are not overlooking iron in your nutritional goals, and have your iron status checked periodically to pick up low iron levels at an early stage.

### Daily recovery

With a twice daily training program, it is not surprising that recovery is regarded as a magic word in triathlon circles. The faster the recovery, the sooner or harder the next session can be. Triathletes often tread precariously along the fine line between hard training and overtraining. During the competitive season, recovery is important for those who want to race each weekend, or to pick up their training straight after each event.

Your peak training diet should supply all the nutrients required for recovery between sessions, with emphasis on fluid strategies (Chapter 1.5) and carbohydrate intake (Chapters 1.3 and 2.2). Chapter 6 has special notes for rapid replacement of fluid and carbohydrate stores after prolonged exercise sessions.

In planning your training schedule, organise the order of sessions to allow maximum recovery time for the specific muscle groups involved in each sport. Also note that hard running causes some muscle fibre damage and requires a longer time to refill muscle glycogen stores. Plan the week accordingly, giving yourself adequate time and extra carbohydrate following intense running sessions or races.

### Preparation for an event

Race preparation depends on the length of the race, the training state of the athlete, and race aspirations. Pre-race strategies are covered in Chapter 4 and should involve preparation of adequate fuel and fluid stores. You may also try to manipulate an empty gut to leave you racing light.

For short events, a well-trained triathlete is able to store sufficient muscle glycogen with a 24–36 hour preparation of rest/taper and a high-carbohydrate diet. If it's your big race for the year, you might like to take a longer taper. Others who are training for longer events later in the season may not want to sacrifice even one day of exercise. Plan your preparation according to your short-term and long-term priorities.

Long course and ultra-distance events challenge muscle glycogen stores and therefore deserve a modified carbohydrate loading preparation. Therefore the last 72 hours should be devoted to glycogen storage, with a rest from exercise and a high-carbohydrate diet. With most races starting early in the morning, the typical pre-race meal is small and light, and eaten on rising about two hours pre-event.

### Food and fluid intake during the race

For sprint races and events up to the Olympic distance, fluid needs are of greatest importance to competitors, and water is probably the most widely used fluid. Race rules generally insist that competitors carry a full bidon (water bottle) on their bikes, and race organisers provide additional fluids at aid stations in the transition areas, and sometimes on the run leg. While those who are out for long hours in the heat of the day are reminded about the need to take in fluids, even top athletes should be warned about the dangers of failing to drink on the bike or run. Chapter 4 explains that moderate fluid loss can reduce performance, and on hot days severe dehydration is a real threat to life and limb. The new drinking pouches consisting of a pressurised sack with a plastic tube fitting along the bike frame to the triathlete's mouth can provide easy access to fluid for those who worry about wasting precious seconds reaching down to the bidon cage.

As events become longer, the advantages of consuming carbohydrate during the race become more obvious. Carbohydrate intake will improve performance in long-course distance and ultra-distance events, by supplying additional fuel sources for trained muscles once glycogen stores have been exhausted (But, you might like to experiment with this in Olympic distance races also). In ultra-distance races, there is usually a well-organised network of aid stations at which athletes are offered a range of food and fluids including sports drinks. See the account of the Ironman race below, and read Chapter 4.7 for guidelines to an well-organised feeding schedule. Most importantly, practise your intended strategies in training.

*Ergogenic aids and dietary supplements*

The past few triathlon seasons have seen a proliferation of supplements and ergogenic aids on the market, many bearing the endorsement of top triathletes. Read Chapter 6 to see which supplements can have an important and useful role in your training and competition, and which products are still awaiting scientific study. Make up your own mind once you have the facts in hand.

PROFILE: VICTOR
*Variety is the spice!*

Victor's friends complained that they never saw him any more—not since triathlon came into his life. Either he was out training or he was in bed early to recover for the next morning's session. There was little point inviting Victor over for dinner—he had become so fussy about his diet that there was little that you could serve him.

From the moment he bought his bike, Victor was hooked on triathlon and searched for any factor to improve his performance. One day while watching *Wide World of Sports* he saw an interview with Dave Scott. When he saw Dave wash his cottage cheese under the tap to remove the last bit of fat, Victor decided it was time for him to clean up his dietary act.

Once a chocolate fiend, he set about eliminating all sources of fat, sugar, salt and alcohol from his diet. He read Pritikin and decided to go one better by becoming a complete vegetarian. The key word, as in training, was discipline. He found that it was amazing how much he could give up, once he put his mind to it. Learning to read food labels was important in case there was some added sugar, fat, or worse still, chemicals. It soon became easier to go without manufactured food, and to cook up a plate of steamed vegetables instead.

Within a month the results were obvious. Gone were those stubborn four kilograms, and Victor felt trim and terrific in training. But by the end of six months another five kilograms was lost, and even Victor agreed that he was looking a bit too thin. Not that it mattered what

he looked like—he felt it was how he rode the bike that was important. However, even that was becoming a problem. Victor found that
his endurance and his recovery were beginning to waver, and that it
was hard to do two solid training days back-to-back. The more he
trained, the worse his times became. It was impossible to ride the
wind trainer for more than an hour—without a comfortable layer of
fat, he found his rear end became too numb on the hard bike seat.
And had the pool forgotten to pay its electricity bill? The water had
become so cold that Victor was shivering between sets of intervals.
He thought of wearing his wet suit to early morning training sessions
to try and ward off another of the colds that seemed to plague him
lately.

It was a delicate problem that finally prompted Victor to seek nutritional advice. Gradually over a period of time, he had developed
gastrointestinal problems. His training partners were complaining about
the constant pit-stops during runs. And nobody wanted to sit on his
wheel when riding, no matter how strong the head wind was. He had
become a one-man environmental hazard!

Victor wrote out a day's menu to show the sports dietitian (see
below) and said, 'It's obviously something wrong that I'm eating. What
else should I cut out of my diet?'

The answer that had eluded Victor, jumped out at the dietitian.
There was no need to eliminate more foods—in fact the process of

---

**Victor describes his daily diet to the dietitian**

---

Before swimming:  2 plain rice cakes (plain—jam and sugar are as bad as honey)

Breakfast:  Large bowl of rolled oats, unprocessed bran, and water (I heard that milk gives
you mucous problems. I used to eat packaged cereals but I'm suspicious of what
they put into them these days)
Pritikin bread + Pritikin jam (when I can get it)
Herbal tea

Morning tea:  Rice cakes—plain
Occasionally Pritikin fruit bread

Lunch:  Large container of salad
Rice cakes
4–5 pieces of fruit
(Sometimes I have a fruit-only lunch: 6–10 pieces)
Plain mineral water
(Are there any fruit juices that are *really* sugar-free?)

Afternoon tea:  I've cut this out to help stop my diarrhea during after-work running sessions

Tea:  Big plate of steamed vegetables
or wholemeal rice with steamed vegetables
or wholemeal pasta with tomato puree sauce
(I have cut out all meats, fish and chicken to eliminate fat totally)
Fruit salad or another bowl of porridge

Supper:  Toasted Pritikin bread with Pritikin sugar-free jam

During long rides:  Water, rice cakes, bananas, dried fruit

elimination was the cause of his present problem. While Victor was to be congratulated for his interest in his diet, his enthusiasm to curb his intake of salt, fat, sugar and food additives had gone too far. The advantages of a varied diet—flexibility, enjoyment and moderation with all nutrients—were lost.

Such a restricted diet was causing a number of problems. For a start, there were too few kilojoules due to the lack of food choices and the bulkiness of meals. Body weight had dropped, probably at the expense of muscle mass and strength, but also to a level of body fat that was no longer healthy.

By eliminating certain foods, Victor had been successful in drastically reducing his fat intake, but had also sacrificed other important nutrients from the same foods—protein from dairy foods and meats, iron and zinc from red meats, and calcium from dairy products. Since he had failed to explore alternative sources of these nutrients from plant food sources, in time it was likely that a nutrient deficiency would occur and further reduce performance.

As for Victor's fear about the chemicals in food, he had overlooked the most sensible approach—a widely varied diet will reduce the risk of overexposure to *any* one food component. The dietitian explained that all substances in food were technically chemicals, and that Victor's diarrhea and flatulence were due to overeating fibre. Clearly, Victor needed to learn about good uses of food—mixing and matching a variety of foods to maximise their valuable features while reducing any less-desirable aspects.

It took a while for Victor to overcome the fear and misconceptions that he had built up about food. But impressed with the arguments in favour of a varied diet, he gradually introduced or re-introduced himself to the great food range around him. He learned how he could still eat many of his favourite foods, but by modifying the type and amount eaten, he could still keep his diet low in fat. He was happy to incorporate animal foods back into his food plans.

Victor became intrigued with clever mixing and matching of foods at meals, and took delight in seeing how many different foods he could combine on his plate. Armed with recipes from the dietitian, he explored different pastas, grains and vegetables, even beans and other legumes. With wholemeal grains and cereals, and plenty of fresh fruit and vegetables, he realised that the fibre content of his diet was already high, so out went the unprocessed bran.

As he became more relaxed with his ability to choose foods well, he became confident about eating out at restaurants and with friends. There were usually a couple of choices on the menu that were suitable, even if he did have to ask the waiter to make some modifications to his order—such as leaving the butter off the bread, or making his cappacino with skim milk. He was also delighted to find that the occasional Mars Bar didn't kill him—in fact it tasted terrific!

Gradually, his gut problems disappeared and his weight and training stamina returned. Most importantly, his friends and training partners no longer needed to avoid him.

PROFILE: GRACE
*A 226-kilometre picnic*

Grace stood on the pier at Kailua-Kona and thought of the race before her. This day had been the focus of her attention for the past six months. Since few people qualify for the Hawaii Ironman World Championship Triathlon she was determined to give her all to the gruelling event: a 3.9km swim, 180km cycle and 42km run. Just to finish would be enough, but Grace also set herself the goal of completing the race with a smile on her face.

Her preparation had left nothing to chance. Once her entry had been confirmed, she began to pick the brains of other triathletes who had competed the Ironman race in previous years. She asked about the food availability in Hawaii—would she be able to follow her usual food plan in the days leading up to the event? How were the aid stations organised at the race itself? What would they be providing to help her meet the massive nutritional challenges on the day?

Her friends assured her that the town of Kailua-Kona would provide her with similar food variety to that in Australia, and that in the days leading up to the event she could look forward to many 'all-you-can-eat' carbo-loading parties. Her race instruction booklet outlined the following aid station plan:

Aid stations:

Bike leg: aid station every 5 miles (8km)

Run leg: aid station every mile (1.6km)

Additional stations at race start and transition areas

Menu:

Water, Coke, Gatorade sports drink, oranges, bananas, guava jelly sandwiches, chocolate-chip cookies

Although there was an opportunity to collect a special provision bag with her own food choices at the half-way mark, Grace decided to stick with the Ironman menu. She read plenty of sports nutrition articles and learned that her priorities would be firstly to keep as well-hydrated as possible, and then to supply herself with a constant intake of carbohydrate—about 50g of carbohydrate per hour was the amount recommended by sports scientists.

The carbohydrate drinks, particularly the sports drinks, seemed the best choice since they could supply both needs simultaneously. Theoretically at least, the drinks should be rapidly emptied from her stomach and quickly transported to her working muscles. Although the solid foods could supply carbohydrate, Grace remembered a couple of occasions when she had eaten during a long run, and had felt uncomfortable with the food sloshing around in her stomach. However, she realised this was personal, since many of her training partners could consume bananas and muesli bars without problems.

Grace bought some Gatorade and started using it in training. She read that on race day she should start drinking this early in the race, and then continue with small amounts at regular intervals. She calculated that an intake of about 800ml per hour would supply her baseline carbohydrate target (50g). Knowing that she should reach an aid station in the bike leg at about 15 minute spacings, this would mean an intake of about 200ml of drink between each. For her, the aid stations in the run leg would be about ten minutes apart, meaning that she should drink perhaps 125–150ml at each. Of course, this would not look after her fluid needs entirely. In the extreme heat in Hawaii she anticipated that she might lose over a litre of sweat per hour. She decided that she would take extra water at each station and drink additional fluid as needed.

The last thing she learned from other triathletes was to be flexible in her plan. What if she got to an aid station and missed the right drink? What if she got hungry? What if she got sick of the taste of the Gatorade? With commonsense, Grace realised that her plan might need to be altered as she went. She might need to drink extra fluid, or as her pace and the day's heat subsided her fluid losses might drop. If she got hungry a small amount of solid food should allay the discomfort. A drink of Coke could give her a 'change of scenery' at times. There was plenty of time over the six months of training to think and experiment.

Grace arrived in Kailua-Kona ten days before the race to acclimatise—to the weather, to the race atmosphere, and to the course itself. The last three days were spent carbo-loading, resting, and drinking plenty of fluid. A light breakfast on rising at 4.30am, and then she found herself at the race start with the other 1199 competitors who shared her own excitement and anticipation.

The race was all that she thought it would be. It was tough—but you don't earn the title of Ironman for nothing! After the swim she stopped briefly in the transition area for a drink, then departed on the bike. With two bidon cages mounted on the frame she was able to keep one bidon of Gatorade and another of water, replacing them alternately at each aid station. She judged her intake to be about 900ml per hour, mostly from Gatorade, and was glad of the extra water to throw over her head at times.

During the run, she alternated her drinks at each aid station—iced water, Gatorade and then Coke. A few orange segments were a refreshing change at times, and at one station she was grateful for a sandwich.

When the finish line loomed ahead, her weary legs felt as if they were running a four-minute mile over the last flood-lit stretch. But from the smile on her face, there was little need to ask if it was all worth while. She didn't feel like drinking a Gatorade cocktail to celebrate, but Grace would remember this race for the rest of ther life—long after the texta colour numbers 'sunburned' into her arms faded.

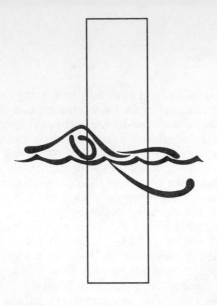

# Swimming

Preparation for elite level swimming begins at an early age, usually around 10–12 years. Typically, the careers of elite swimmers also finish early, at around 20 years for women and 25 for males. There is now reason to see this as mental or lifestyle burn out rather than physiological burnout. In recent years there have been many noted swimmers who have returned from retirement to swim again in open or Masters level swimming. Many have been able to improve or duplicate their earlier performances.

At the Olympic level, swimming events are held in a number of strokes (freestyle, breaststroke, backstroke and butterfly), over distances ranging from 50m to 1500m. Long-distance swimming, in which a swimmer may complete an individual time-trial or group race in open water, has a much smaller following but was included in the World Swimming Championships for the first time in 1991. Long distance swimming races may involve distances from five to 50km, and are often held in the waterways between two famous landpoints—for example the English Channel. This chapter will be devoted to Olympic-event swimming.

## Training

By the time they are 12 or 13, many swimmers have already taken on a serious commitment to training. Typically, training sessions are held in the early morning (e.g. 5–7am) and then in the late afternoon (e.g. 4–6pm) to fit around school or work commitments. The number of training sessions undertaken by a swimmer will vary, depending on their age, the events for which they are preparing, and the stage of the season. Typically, six to twelve sessions can be undertaken each week, with the distance covered in each session ranging from 1000–2000 metres of quality work for a sprinter in a taper phase, to ten kilometres for a distance swimmer in the base phase of training. The heaviest workloads can chalk up 100km of swimming each week, with twice-daily sessions adding up to almost six hours of training per day. At the club or school level, training commitments are considerably smaller than this, and swimmers may not train all year round.

Swimming training varies with the phase of the season, to include an initial aerobic endurance base, followed by various anaerobic training sessions where single or multi-effort intervals are swum at different percentages of maximal work output. Heart rate and blood lactate levels are measured to monitor the various types of work-outs. In addition to these sessions, swimmers commonly include weight training, typically three sessions per week. Some swimmers also undertake aerobic land training, such as running or cycling, to help reduce body-fat levels. Such a program calls heavily on muscle glycogen stores, and swimmers who fail to replenish their stores on a daily basis may be unable to complete such high-intensity sessions.

Peaking for competition involves a period of tapering with a reduced training load. Swimmers who compete in a number of competitions over the year may not fully prepare for them all, and may concentrate on peaking for one or two major competitions.

### Competition

It takes about 25 seconds for an elite swimmer to race over 50 metres and about 15 minutes to complete 1500m—making swimming a highly anaerobic sport with aerobic metabolism becoming more important as the race distance increases. Muscle fuel stores will not be depleted even over a 1500m swim, with the main source of fatigue being a build-up of lactate and the accompanying products of anaerobic metabolism.

Swim meets are usually held over three to five days, with swimmers typically competing in heats in the mornings and the final of that event in the evening. In minor carnivals, swimmers may enter a large number of events and be required to swim two or three times in one day, with 20 minutes to several hours between events. At major competitions, only exceptional swimmers will enter more than three events. Light warm-ups are completed prior to each competition session and training is often scheduled for non-competition days.

### Physical characteristics

Swimmers are noted for their upper body muscle development—back, chest, arms and shoulders—they are also usually tall, particularly the sprinters. Since swimmers are required to move their own body mass through water, low body fat is an advantage. However, the buoyancy of water makes body fat less of a disadvantage than it is on dry land. In fact, some body fat in the right distribution can enhance floatation. Swimmers specialising in the longer events often have higher body-fat levels than the sprinters. Open water long-distance swimmers often carry large amounts of body fat to provide buoyancy, and insulation against the cold.

**Typical physique (elite Australian Olympic swimmers)**

|  | Male | Female |
|---|---|---|
| Height | 181–193cm | 168–177cm |
| Weight | 72–86kg | 57–67kg |
| Skinfolds | 43–57mm | 53–77mm |

## Other comments

Many top swimmers are in their teens, and the physical changes experienced with puberty may help to explain an interesting observation—male swimmers are more likely to have trouble eating enough kilojoules to meet energy needs, while female swimmers struggle to lose body fat. This is because male adolescence is a period of heavy growth and muscular development, requiring high energy support, while females undergo hormonal changes which promote an increase in body fat. For males then, the addition of an intense training program means that total energy needs can reach an almost unbelievable level, while the female swimmer, despite equally strenuous training, works uphill against the hormonal messages to lay down fat.

The long hours of training place a heavy restriction on a swimmer's lifestyle, limiting the social and recreational activities typical of teenagers. This can either reduce the opportunities to eat in a busy daily schedule, or conversely, raise the importance of eating for comfort or entertainment value. Thus, both underweight and overweight problems are common in swimming.

Access to food can also be an issue at swimming carnivals and meets, with many swimmers travelling away from home to compete. Hotels and 'athlete villages' may provide unsuitable food choices and the lack of supervision may further encourage poor eating patterns.

## Common nutrition issues

### Daily recovery

Strenuous daily training calls for a high-energy, high-carbohydrate diet. American physiologist Professor David Costill conducted a study on a squad of male swimmers who suddenly doubled their training load. While some of the squad adapted to this increase, the other swimmers experienced difficulty—complaining of fatigue and muscle soreness. Analysis of their diets showed that the first group had automatically increased their carbohydrate intake to match the increased cost of training, while the other group had not made this adaptation. Muscle glycogen levels of the second group were significantly lower.

This observation is explained in the notes on recovery, and is illustrated in Figure 5.1 (Chapter 5). Read Chapters 1.3 and 2.2 for information about good habits with carbohydrate foods to promote daily recovery in training. In Grant's story below, help was needed to make the carbohydrate kilojoules compact. A bulky diet requires more time to chew than most busy athletes can afford.

## Fluid needs in training

Swimmers can churn up and down the pool for hours—often in the steamy environment of a heated indoor pool, and occasionally outdoors in the late afternoon heat. This can lead to large sweat losses, which are not obvious when you are already wet. Hopping out of the pool to get a drink is not always possible. Smart swimming coaches now insist that swimmers bring their own water bottles to the edge of the pool. Drinking during rest periods or between sets will help you to train better.

## High energy requirements

The energy cost of training, particularly when added to energy needs for growth, can mean a very high total energy requirement. This is typically an issue for male swimmers, and can be compounded by the lack of the time in the day to eat. Chapter 3.7 deals with hints to help a swimmer achieve a high energy intake, by increasing the number of meals and snacks in the day and making use of energy-dense foods. Planning ahead to have a portable and compact food supply can win the battle for you.

## Weight loss and the typical female swimmer

Female swimmers fight a notorious battle to keep body-fat measurements down at their desired levels. Despite heavy training they often complain that they do not seem to burn the expected kilojoules. Not only can this become frustrating, but the constant focus on diet and weight loss can mean that thinking about food almost takes over the day. Everything revolves around food—entertainment, comfort when upset or depressed, celebration or commiseration. It can become a vicious circle. You eat because you are upset. Your skinfolds go up, making you more upset, so you have something to eat to make you feel better. And so on.

While it may seem unfair that male swimmers can eat twice as much as you, or that some girls in your squad can eat what they like without dreading the mirror or the skinfold tests, if you concentrate on yourself instead of comparing yourself to others, you will probably find that you *can* improve your lot. Read Chapter 3, about setting a body-fat target that is realistic for *you*, and then committing yourself to a long-term fat-loss program that is right for *your* situation. Above all, set yourself the goal to become comfortable with your body shape and your enjoyment of food.

### Eating disorders

There are many reports that female swimmers are at high risk of developing eating disorders—or more likely, that many swimmers resort to unhealthy techniques such as self-induced vomiting (bulimia), and the use of diuretics and laxatives. Most often these practices are used as a short-term solution to weight-loss problems. The problem is that they do not solve, or even attack, the real problem. In most cases the issue is overconcern about body fat and food, and a poor self-image. The body-fat problem itself is usually secondary, and in some cases wildly exaggerated. However, the unhealthy eating behaviour can add to your woes by directly impairing performance and health.

Read Chapter 3 for a sensible approach to goal-setting, with body-fat targets and fat-loss program. The best help may come from talking things over with professionals—a sports psychologist who can help you to restore your self-confidence, and a dietitian who can support you to get back into healthy training nutrition.

### Iron status

Strenuous daily training places a stress on body iron stores. While swimming doesn't cause the same physical trauma as running, one study of swimmers reported that red blood cells were damaged by the continual impact of turbulent water. Even if this is not a widespread occurrence, female swimmers on weight-loss diets are at risk of a low iron intake. Read Chapter 2.5 to learn about good sources of iron. Have your iron status checked regularly when you are in heavy training.

### Competition nutrition

Muscle glycogen stores can be filled by 24 hours of a high-carbohydrate diet and exercise taper (see Chapter 4). Be aware, if you are doing a longer taper, that you may need to reduce your total energy intake to match the reduced workload, otherwise you may suddenly gain body fat.

Since events can be held at various times of the day, careful planning of the pre-event meal may be needed (see Chapter 4). This may be a challenge if you are away from home, and it often helps to bring some food supplies of your own.

Between events you should replenish fluid levels and top up carbohydrate stores. If you have more than three hours between events a light carbohydrate meal might be eaten in comfort. Liquid meal supplements (Exceed Sports Nutrition Supplement or Sustagen) provide another alternative. Where there is only a short interval between races, drink a carbohydrate-containing fluid—a sports drink, fruit juice or soft drink should be suitable (Chapter 5).

### Communal eating—the athlete's dining hall

A communal dining hall can be a culture shock to young swimmers, especially when being away from home is a new experience. This situation may be faced on swimming camps, at the athletes' village during big competitions, or by residents of the Australian Institute of Sport. For many, the change from the family meal table can provide a huge challenge, and bad decisions may be made with food. This can result in both short-term consequences (perhaps upsetting competition performance) and long-term problems (upsetting training nutrition goals). The dining hall story below illustrates that special tactics can be used to ensure that food is well chosen.

PROFILE: GRANT
*Chewing through the carbos*

A lot of Grant's day was spent staring at the black line on the bottom of the pool, especially since his squad had increased their training to twelve sessions a week. At first he had coped with the extra training load, but by the end of the second month he was feeling fatigued. Not only were his times beginning to drop off, but his school work had started to get on top of him as well. To cap it all off, his weight seemed to be going down and he could not really afford to lose any more body fat. Grant's mother encouraged him to eat a larger serve of meat at the evening meal, but by this time of the night he was often too tired to do more than pick at it.

A sports dietitian listened to Grant's story and examined his diet. She advised him that additional kilojoules were needed to cover the extra training, but that carbohydrate foods were the most important source of the energy for training. Chronic depletion of muscle glycogen stores were the likely cause of his current fatigue problems. At 80kg, a daily intake of 700–800g of carbohydrate was a reasonable target, and his present diet lagged considerably behind that.

They examined a list of carbohydrate foods together, and Grant found that they were all foods he liked to eat—bread, breakfast cereals, fruit, potatoes, rice and pasta. However, the problem was how to fit more of them into his day. He already left the meal table feeling too tired or too full to eat another mouthful. Listening to Grant's typical daily meal plan, the dietitian pointed out that he relied only on three meals per day—breakfast, hastily eaten in the car on the way from the pool to school, lunch, juggled between school activities, and a late evening meal at home.

The solution lay in increasing the *number* of meals rather than the *size*, and in choosing carbohydrate foods which were portable and easy to eat. Planning and preparation would be needed to have the right food on hand at school and during travelling times. Liquid meals, both homemade 'smoothies' and the commercial preparations, would come in handy, supplying kilojoules and carbohydrates with little bulk. These could be drunk in addition to meals, or as a snack between meals, without making him feel uncomfortable at training. The following plan was suggested:

**Sample high carbohydrate (high-energy) eating plan for Grant (swimmer)**

Breakfast: Brought from home and eaten at the pool after training:
2 large bowls of mixed cereals (untoasted muesli, Weetbix, Sustain etc) plus milk, chopped banana or other fresh fruit.
Fruit juice—500ml

Recess: 2 X 250ml packs of Sustagen Gold
Large piece of muesli slice or wholemeal scones
Grab-pack of mixed dried fruits

Lunch: 3 rolls, with salad and meat/egg/chicken/cheese
2 small cartons of fruit-flavoured yoghurt
Fruit juice

After school (on way to training):
250ml can of Exceed Sports Nutrition Supplement

After training (on the way home in the car):
Fruit juice or sports drink

Dinner (waiting for him when he got home):
Large serve of rice/pasta/potatoes
Lean fish/chicken/lean meat
Vegetables or salad
Bread or bread rolls
Fruit juice

Before bed: Milkshake or fruit smoothie with skim milk, fruit (banana, strawberries, etc.), icecream and extra skim milk powder.

Other snacks (weekends): Fruit or fresh fruit salad, crumpets, muffins, pancakes

This eating plan would increase Grant's intake to 800–900g of carbohydrate each day, and 21 000–23 000 kilojoules (5000–5500 cals). The dietitian also pointed out that this pattern allowed Grant to begin eating carbohydrate foods or drinks as soon as training was over.

This way muscle glycogen storage would be activated as quickly as possible.

Within three weeks Grant reported a new feeling of energy at training, and a weight gain of a kilogram. This eating program certainly requires some planning and organisation, but with his new lease of life, Grant has plenty of enthusiasm.

PROFILE: ANGELA
*Eating in a communal dining hall—special tactics for a special situation*

By the time Angela had returned from the Commonwealth Games she had gained over two kilograms. Her coach at home was half expecting it. He had heard of other swimmers going to the Institute of Sport and gaining four kilograms in the first two months, seemingly all body fat. His own daughters at boarding school seemed to have gained weight each time they came home for term holidays, although his son complained that at his University college there was never enough to eat.

Most people who eat in institutions, whether it be a boarding school, a hospital or the Olympic village for athletes have definite views about the food. Common themes are: 'there's no variety'; 'all the goodness is cooked out of it'; 'it's fattening—you'll put on weight'; 'there's never enough to eat—weight just drops off'.

Dining rooms specially set up for athletes, such as the dining hall at the Australian Institute of Sport, or the cafeterias at Games' villages, are definitely not guilty of these charges. In addition to serving massive volumes of food, and staying open for long hours to cater for the various schedules of the athletes, these dining rooms pay particular attention to the nutritional needs of athletes. It is the athlete who is ultimately responsible for what goes into their mouths. In most cases when a situation of poor nutrition is closely examined, the real problem is found to be what the athlete is choosing—not the food opportunities themselves.

Most people are accustomed to a family meal environment, or to cooking for themselves. In these situations they get used to having one food choice at a time, and despite the fact that they think they eat a variety of meals, they probably stick to a handful of favourite recipes, with only an occasional change. In any case, it is all very familiar and under control.

The sudden switch to a communal cafeteria-style dining hall is a culture shock to most athletes. The following new features and challenges are thrown at you:

- Great quantities and many different choices of food. You can serve yourself as much as you like from a never-ending supply, and there are so many nice things to try. Many athletes find that under these circumstances, it is easy to eat more than usual, and more than they need.

- Limited access to food outside designated eating times. If the dining hall is only open at certain times, athletes with enormous energy needs may not be able to consume sufficient food at the customary three sittings. This may lead to weight loss in these athletes.

- Different and unusual foods. It can be challenging to find a new set of foods and meals awaiting you. You may be reluctant to experiment when it comes to trying new foods, or maybe you are unsure of their nutritional value. This can lead to weight loss or failure to meet nutritional goals.

- Lack of supervision. Many athletes come unstuck when they first move to the dining hall and find that Mum is no longer around to make eat them their vegetables.

- Distraction from other athletes. Surrounded by the eating habits of a large group of people, you may find it hard to concentrate on your own nutritional goals. And, given the competitive nature of athletes, it isn't surprising that official and unofficial 'eating competitions' can take place.

- Eating for entertainment. An athlete may not have much time and scope for leisure activities during the day. If the dining hall becomes the meeting place, a lot of extra food can be demolished in the name of relaxation and recreation.

Faced with these challenges, the athlete must develop special skills and tactics to use the dining hall to its optimum potential. The following hints will help you make good decisions:

---

## HINTS FOR EATING WELL IN A CAFETERIA-STYLE EATING HALL

- Develop the right attitude. The food is not 'fattening' or 'bad for you'. How you select from the food choices will determine whether you meet your nutritional goals.

- Treat the dining room like a restaurant. If there is no written menu, take the time to survey the choices before you commit yourself to a queue. Make a decision about what you will choose for that meal and then serve yourself. (Don't get into the line and keep adding more food to your plate as you pass by each dish). Make certain that you meet your nutritional goals, rather than stumble on them by accident.

---

- Don't be distracted by the other foods you have not chosen for this meal. There will be other opportunities to try the things you missed today.

- Although the food choices available may generally reflect the guidelines for peak training nutrition, you may still have to exercise restraint or modify food choices to fully meet your goals. You may have the option of skim milk rather than full cream, or to cut the remaining fat from the meat. Make the best of these opportunities.

- Allow yourself some flexibility for special foods—but choose treats well with your nutritional goals in mind.

- Don't concern yourself with the amount and types of foods that other athletes consume. Stick to what is right for you and realise that athletes vary with their nutritional needs.

- Remove yourself from the food environment once you have finished eating. Don't leave yourself exposed to boredom eating.

- If your energy needs go beyond the meal opportunities offered at the dining hall, take a snack for later on—a sandwich, some fruit or yoghurt are good choices.

- If needed, make use of any opportunities to seek expert dietary advice or to have special services arranged for you. There is often a dietitian for any queries or problems. They may also be able to arrange extra food or nutritional supplements to boost inadequate energy intake.

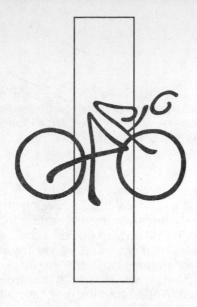

# Cycling

Competitive cycling includes the separate sports of track and road cycling, both with distinct amateur and professional divisions, and the growing sport of mountain bike racing. This chapter will deal with track and road cycling events.

Cycle races range from sprint races lasting about ten seconds to stage races, such as the Tour de France, covering around 4000km over three weeks. They include individual events and team events and involve not only physiological demands, but a mastery of technique and tactics, as well as great courage. The variety of distances and types of races has resulted in the specialisation of cyclists into events which have similar demands.

Track cycling is undertaken on a sloped track at a velodrome, and ranges from the sprint event to the 50km point score race (basically a distance event). Other events include team and individual pursuits, the kilometre time trial and the Keiren. Track events rely on a range of capabilities from sprint power to speed endurance, and anaerobic energy production plays a vital role in most races.

Road races may be held over a number of stages (days), or as single day events. Other events include time trials (both team and individual) and the criterium (a race of varying numbers of laps around a circuit of roads). Races vary in distance from a couple of kilometres for some criteriums, to individual stages of 250km or more, and thousands of kilometres in multi-day events. Road cycling is primarily concerned with strength endurance and endurance, although anaerobic capacity may be called upon in breakaways, hill climbing and all-out sprints to the line.

*117*

In some countries, e.g. Australia, the road and track seasons are held at different times, making it possible for cyclists to compete in both sports. However, the specialist nature of various events means that very few cyclists excel in both areas.

### Training

In the off-season, training consists primarily of road cycling to build up aerobic fitness, and weight training to develop strength. For cyclists who concentrate solely on track events, strength training is of considerable importance in building up power. Leading up to and during the competitive season, road work and weight training are reduced in favour of specific track training, with the emphasis on quality rather than quantity. During these sessions both anaerobic power and endurance are developed. Weight training may be continued throughout the season, but sessions are less frequent.

Road cyclists do most of their training on the road, and training distances vary with the time of the year. At the elite level, training involves at least daily sessions, with weekly distances tallying 400–1000km. At the height of the season in Europe, cyclists may do little training since they are continually racing—thanks to a packed race calendar and a selection of stage races.

### Competition

Track cycling competitions, depending on their size, may vary from single-day to multi-day meets. Time trials and handicap races are one-off events, while the points score, the sprints and pursuits involve heats and finals. In the latter case, a competitor may be required to race more than once on the same day. Since most events are sprint-based, the depletion of fuel stores is generally not an issue.

Road cycling races are run as one-off events, and become more physiologically and nutritionally challenging as the duration of the race increases. In general, races of 100km require attention to fluid and carbohydrate intake during the event—a practical consideration for both competitors and race organisers. Races vary with their rules and support for intake during the event itself. Some organisers provide feed station(s) at intervals along the route, others require competitors to carry their own race food and drinks or to organise their own support crew. In stage races, accommodation and meals are often part of the race package, although many teams will provide additional back-up.

### Physical characteristics

Physical characteristics vary between cyclists specialising in different types of races. In general, cyclists are muscular and lean, with increasing muscularity amongst track sprinters and increasing leanness amongst the distance competitors. Body fat levels of cyclists are low, particularly in the case of road cyclists where hill-climbing requires a high power-to-weight ratio.

**Typical physique (elite track cyclists)**

|  | Male | Female |
| --- | --- | --- |
| Height | 178–182cm | 162–170cm |
| Weight | 72–80kg | 54–62kg |
| Skinfold sum | 36–50mm | 58–92mm |

**Typical physique (elite road cyclists)**

|  | Male |  |
| --- | --- | --- |
| Height | 174–187cm | Sufficient data not yet |
| Weight | 67–80kg | available for females. |
| Skinfold sum | 35–57mm |  |

## Common nutrition issues

### Training nutrition

Training for cycling, particularly distance road events, can be time and energy-consuming. The long kilometres and hours of training undertaken by elite cyclists call for a high energy diet—high in protein, vitamins and minerals, and high in carbohydrate for muscle fuel stores (read Chapters 1 and 2 for a discussion of the optimum training diet). Daily recovery between heavy training sessions requires a high total carbohydrate intake, but also clever timing of meals and snacks to enhance muscle glycogen restoration. Chapter 5 explains that a carbohydrate snack immediately following a long training session, will kick-start muscle glycogen synthesis and prepare fuel stores for tomorrow's (or this afternoon's) training session.

A pattern of frequent meals and snacks may also be handy for making sure that total energy and carbohydrate needs are met (Chapters 2.7 and 3.7). With the magnitude and bulkiness of food requirements, it can be hard to live on three meals a day. A dietary study of elite cyclists estimated their average daily energy intake at over 26 000 kilojoules (6200 Cals). This was only made possible by a pattern of constant 'grazing' over the day. Imagine trying to eat this as three 8000 kilojoule feasts every day—it would be the equivalent of three Christmas dinners.

Iron status may be an issue for female cyclists—read Chapter 2.5

and see how a high iron intake can be compatible with a high carbo-hydrate diet.

### Body-fat levels

Most endurance cyclists take care of their body-fat levels through heavy training. In some situations, particularly in the case of female athletes or athletes coming back after a break, there may be an additional effort needed to help shed the spare tyres. See Chapter 3 for a discussion of sensible and successful methods of weight loss.

### Food and fluid needs during long rides

Whether in training or in competition, cyclists ride over distances that challenge their fluid and fuel levels. In hot weather and when working hard, sweat losses can be high. Of course you may not notice this since the sweat evaporates quickly in the wind. Nevertheless, moderate to severe dehydration will result in performance losses—obviously critical on race day, but also a disadvantage to good training.

Endurance performance is also effected by the depletion of body carbohydrate stores—through the depletion of muscle glycogen stores and/or low blood glucose levels. The heavy 'dead' legs that some cyclists experience are probably due to low muscle glycogen levels in the quads. Meanwhile, 'the bonk' or 'hunger flat' are more likely to be the result of blood sugar decline—notice how quickly you can pick up after eating some carbohydrate. Cyclists seem more susceptible to low blood sugar levels than other distance athletes such as runners. Some individuals are particularly susceptible—you may have observed that other riders can go all day on very little food, while more than 50km without a banana will see you falling off the bike.

Clearly, good performance will mean looking after fluid and carbo-hydrate intake during exercise. A cyclist can be more self-reliant than other athletes, in that food and drinks can be carried on the bike—food in the pockets of a cycling jersey or in a 'bum bag', and fluid in bidons (bottles) carried in cages mounted on the bike frame. Because of this, road races are less organised in providing aid stations to competitors than a running marathon would be. Depending on the history and tradition of the race, or the traffic safety rules under which it operates, a cycle race may provide little or no outside aid to competitors. Some races allow riders to have individual handlers to supply food and drinks during the race, but other events place competitors behind the nutritional eight-ball by allowing only what can be carried by the rider themselves. Some of these races can be over distances up to 260km.

Clearly, both cyclists and race organisers need to update their sports nutrition knowledge. Read Chapter 4.7 for the principles of endurance exercise intake. As a rule of thumb, carbohydrate intake should be organised for rides over 100km, and fluid needs will vary both with the distance and the weather conditions. Be prepared, according to the race rules, to take your own supplies, and to supplement these where allowable from aid stations (official or individual). Carbohydrate intake needs to start *before* you hit a hunger flat. Again, a rule of thumb is to start to eat by 40km into the race. As outlined in Chapter 4.7, an aggressive intake of about 50g of carbohydrate per hour is needed— perhaps even more in the last stages of a race when body carbohydrate stores are very low.

On the bike, a range of solid and liquid forms of sustenance are possible, and indeed a wide range of foods have been successfully used during long races. While sports drinks provide state-of-the-art exercise intake, it may be difficult to transport sufficient liquid on the bike for the whole race. Two bidon cages should be mounted for long races in hot weather, particularly when no outside aid is allowed. A one-litre bidon in each can then provide a reasonable intake of fluid and carbohydrate (two litres of fluid and 140g of carbohydrate from a sports drink with a 7 per cent carbohydrate concentration). Extra fluid may be needed on very hot days and for very long races. If required, extra carbohydrate food can also be carried in your jersey—bananas, dried fruit, Power Bars and muesli bars are popular choices. As discussed in Chapter 4.7, practise in training so that your competition plans are fool-proof.

A final word on training—good fluid and fuel practices will not only prepare you for your competition strategies, but they will also improve your training form. It is tempting to go out on four-hour training rides with a single bidon of fluid, and not want to interrupt your rhythm by stopping to refill the bottle. While you may not always 'blow up', you may spend the rest of the day with a headache and fail to bounce back for your next training session. Try not to let dehydration go beyond one or two kilograms of your body weight.

*Competition nutrition and the pre-event meal*

For most racing, especially track racing, a well-trained athlete should be capable of taking in adequate fuel stores with 24–36 hours of preparation. See Chapter 4.2 for details.

The pre-event meal is important for topping up stores and for making the athlete feel comfortable during the race. Choose a light meal or snack according to the guidelines in Chapter 4.4. Most people consider cyclists are not worried by a stomach of food to the same extent as a runner—after all, the food doesn't get joggled around so much. However, if you are crouched over your bars in a streamlined position, then a full stomach can be uncomfortable and can interfere with your breathing. If this is a problem for you, try a liquid meal supplement such as Sustagen or Exceed Sports Nutrition Supplement. This is a good way of taking in low-bulk sustenance.

### Endurance competition—carbohydrate loading

Distance races should be tackled with full muscle glycogen stores. Where a weekly program of road racing is underway, it is not possible to undertake a carbohydrate loading schedule 3 days prior to each race. Good recovery nutrition will help to replenish carbohydrate stores throughout the training week, but there may not be adequate time to fully store muscle glycogen before the race. This will place more emphasis on carbohydrate intake practices during the race.

Of course, for very important races, you may like to reorganise your training and racing schedule to allow for a longer race preparation. See Chapter 4.3 for details of a full carbohydrate loading schedule.

### Multi-stage races—the challenge of recovery

Whether in recreational bike tours or in important professional stages races, many cyclists undertake a schedule of successive-day riding, with individual stages up to 200km and events lasting up to three weeks. These events place enormous stress on the fuel and fluid reserves of the athlete, with the carry-over effect from each day's riding being important. As well as looking after needs during each day's stage, a successful athlete should undertake strategies to assist recovery between days. The main factor of success is not being the best on any one day, but being able to do it again tomorrow. This was highlighted by the feat of Greg Lemond, who in the 1990 Tour de France race became the first rider to win the Tour without having won a single stage along the way.

Recovery nutrition is covered in Chapter 5, with discussion of fluid and carbohydrate replenishment, and in the case of long tours, the need for adequate total nutrient intake. From a practical point of view, nutritional arrangements for multi-day events may be left up to individual competitors or teams, or they may be included in the overall organisation of the event. Often, accommodation and meals are included in the race or tour package and can vary from camp sites and army cooking, to hotel hospitality.

The disadvantages of relying on event organisation include unsuitable food, reliance on the event time-table rather than a time-table that provides for your needs or strategies, and the business of competing with lots of people for the same food. You may be safer to cater partly or fully for your needs—especially if the race organisation is unfamiliar to you, or if your nutritional needs are crucial to good performance. It doesn't hurt to bring some of your own supplies, especially the specific foods and drinks that are part of your race and post-race eating strategies.

Professional teams in important races will often come with a full back-up team and an aggressive nutrition plan. The Tour de France is perhaps the best known multi-stage cycle race, providing riders with an enormous challenge to their riding skills and nutritional knowledge. See the account below to see how the champions survive.

PROFILE
*The Tour de France*

The Tour de France is no picnic—4000km in 20-odd days over some of the most rugged mountain terrain in Europe. Yet eating and drinking, especially on the bike, plays a crucial role in allowing the cyclists to perform well, and for that matter, even to finish the race.

Recently some Dutch physiologists, lead by Professor Wim Saris, conducted an extensive study of this race, following the fortunes of five male cyclists from one of the leading professional teams. Daily energy expenditure was estimated, with the cost of each day's cycling being taken from the detailed descriptions of each stage. Body weight and body fat was checked over the period, and cyclists kept a record of all food and fluid intake over the race.

The first and most remarkable result was the total energy expenditure estimated for the race—with an average daily energy expenditure of 25 400 kilojoules (6060 Cals). The heaviest day of exercise was estimated to cost 32 700 kJ (7800 Cals), and on the one rest day, energy expenditure was estimated to drop below 13 000 kJ (3100 Cals). Despite this energy output, there were only minor changes reported in body weight and body fat over the three-week period. And indeed the estimated energy intake from food, drinks and supplements was reported at a daily average of 24 700 kJ (5900 Cals). The riders did very well in balancing their energy needs over this period, and data suggested that they managed to balance intake and expenditure remarkably well on a daily basis. This was important, since with the large amounts required to be eaten it would be hard to catch up from one day to the next if intake fell behind. There is only so much that you can put into your stomach each day!

A summary of total dietary intake over the race is presented in the following table. Carbohydrate intake was well looked after, making up over 60 per cent of total food intake. The cyclists churned through 12–13g of carbohydrate per kilogram of body mass per day—further evidence of the remarkable work output during the race. Protein intake was more than adequate, supplying about 15 per cent of total energy during the period, or an intake of over 3g/kg body mass/day. Fat intake, supplying about 23 per cent of energy intake, was well below the typical Western dietary ratio.

**Average daily intake of Tour de France cyclists**

| | |
|---|---|
| Energy | 24 300 KJ/day (5800 Cals) |
| Carbohydrate | 849g/day = 61% of energy<br>= 12.3g/kg/day |
| Protein | 217g/day = 15% of energy<br>= 3.1g/kg/day |
| Fat | 147g/day = 23% of energy |
| Water | 6.7 litres/day |

Vitamin and mineral intakes were above requirements, both on the basis of recommended dietary intake levels and from blood measurements of micronutrient status. Not only did these nutrients come from food intake, but from fortified liquid formulas (such as carbohydrate loading and liquid meal supplements) and from additional vitamin supplements as well. As would be expected from sweat loss needs, fluid intake was high—an average of 6.7 litres per day per cyclist.

So what did the cyclists eat? The range of foodstuffs listed included sweet cakes (perhaps contributing more fat than the cyclists realised), pasta, bread and breakfast cereals, with high-protein foods including meats, dairy products and eggs. An important contribution to both carbohydrate and energy intake was made by carbohydrate-rich drinks—soft drinks, and more particularly sports drinks, liquid meal supplements and high-carbohydrate 'carbo-loader' formulas. About a third of total carbohydrate intake was provided by these drinks—obviously an advantage in terms of compact and digestible energy.

It is also of interest to note that a substantial part of the day's intake was consumed while actually on the bike. Nearly half the day's energy and nearly 60 per cent of total carbohydrate intake was consumed during the race, presumably thanks to the carbohydrate liquids. An average of four litres of fluid was also consumed while riding.

Thus our cyclists seem to have made good use of sports nutrition information, using special sports products to boost energy, carbohydrate, and total nutrient intake in a compact form. Intake during the race seemed aggressive and designed to avoid dehydration and fuel depletion, and hopefully post-exercise eating was timed to begin rapid recovery at the end of each day.

The human body is a remarkable engine to be able to tackle such a sustained high-intensity workload, and deserves the very best in fuel and maintenance nutrients.

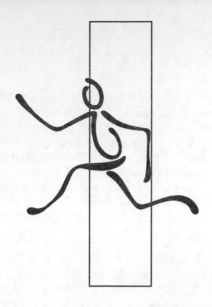

# Distance running

Distance runners compete over a variety of race lengths most commonly 10km, 15km, half marathon (21.1km) and the marathon (42.2km). While there is a 10 000m track event, most distance running is done as road races or cross-country runs. 'Fun runs' of various lengths attract community participation, recreational runners joining with elite and club-level runners.

Ultradistance races such as 50mile, 100km and 100mile events are not included in the Olympic Games or World Championships, and generally do not attract a large following, particularly at the recreational level. Exceptions to this are races such as the South African 'Comrades' run—a race of 90km which attracts a field of 12 000 competitors each year.

Distance runners mature with age, requiring years of base training to build up to the program of an elite runner. Consequently, most elite competitors are aged from their mid-twenties to late thirties. At a recreational level, running is a great leveller, and you would expect to find both teenagers and seventy-year-olds competing in the same fun run.

### Training

At the recreational level, many runners train primarily for fitness or health, and compete in a number of fun runs, and perhaps a marathon, each year. Daily training sessions might add up to a weekly distance of 50km, perhaps peaking at 80–100km before a marathon.

Elite distance runners typically run up to 200km per week, with two training sessions per day. Some runners include water running and weight training in their programs, but this is the exception rather than the rule, and has traditionally been associated with rehabilitation of injuries. A typical training week includes different types of sessions, each with a specific physiological emphasis. Sessions include longer slow runs for aerobic endurance, with intense continuous runs, fartlek or 'speed play' sessions and track (interval) work all undertaken to improve anaerobic capacity and speed.

### Competition

The elite runner may compete in a number of races of varying distance each year, with a few key events being chosen for full preparation and peaking. Many will compete weekly over a season of road races (usually summer) or cross-country runs (usually winter), treating each race as a hard training session. Marathon runners are unlikely to compete more than once or twice a year over this distance.

Events in hot weather are usually held in the early morning to avoid the heat, while cross-country events may be held on winter afternoons. Races are normally held as a once-off competition, i.e. without heats or qualifiers. Relay or stage races are sometimes held, requiring competitors to run a series of 6–10km legs, often with only a short recovery time in between. In international events such as the Olympic Games, some runners will contest both the 10 000m track event and the marathon, with the races being separated by a number of days.

Distance running is predominantly an aerobic activity, with elite athletes running from under 30 minutes (10km) to just over two hours (the marathon). Recreational runners can take up to twice as long to complete the same distance, and sometimes even longer. Races above 30km will probably challenge the usual carbohydrate storage capacity of most runners, and steps will need to be taken to increase or extend muscle glycogen stores.

### Physical characteristics

Distance runners typically carry low body-fat levels—an advantage when you have to carry your body weight over many kilometres. In fact, most elite runners have low total body weights, being small in stature and lightly muscled, particularly in the upper body.

**Typical physique (elite distance runner)**

|  | Male | Female |
| --- | --- | --- |
| Height | 172–182cm | not available |
| Weight | 59–71kg | not available |
| Skinfolds | 29–39mm | not available |

### Other comments

Distance running has for many years attracted the attention of sports scientists. It is a good sport to study, being both popular and predictable—a marathon is always 42.2km, whereas every football match is literally a new ball game. Not only have nutritional and physiological issues been well researched, but the results enjoy good coverage in the popular running magazines.

Thus runners are generally well-educated about their sport. Many recreational runners have read about carbo-loading or what to drink during a marathon, and exercise physiologists, such as Dave Costill and Tim Noakes, are often as well-known as the top runners themselves. Of course, not all the scientific information is understood or turned into good practices, but at least runners have the expectation that scientific approaches to nutrition can aid their performance.

### Common nutrition issues

*Recovery and carbohydrate—the amount and the timing*

Daily and twice daily training sessions call for recovery strategies, especially when two hard sessions are held back-to-back. Even a recreational runner may find that the typical Western diet does not provide sufficient fuel for marathon training. In fact the first time many runners hit the wall is during their first weeks of big training mileage, due to a gradual process of failing to restore muscle glycogen levels.

Recovery will aided both by the amount and timing of the carbohydrate. Read Chapter 5. Chapters 1.3 and 2.2 will guide you to estimate your daily carbohydrate requirements and build in the dietary habits to achieve your carbohydrate intake goals.

The timing of carbohydrate is crucial for recovery after long, hard training sessions or races. Not only are your muscles depleted of carbohydrate, but running also causes some damage to muscle fibres, which will delay glycogen recovery. Carbohydrate intake immediately after the session or the race will let the muscle take advantage of their most rapid recovery time. Don't leave it too long.

*Low body-fat levels*

The low body-fat levels of elite distance runners are typically a result of well-chosen parents and high-volume training. However some runners, both elite and recreational, need additional help to reduce body-fat levels.

The first step is to set a realistic target—a body-fat level that is part of good health as well as good performance, and a body-fat level that can be achieved and maintained with a healthy diet and a sensible workload. Read about this in Chapter 3.

### Females, fat and food disorders

For some runners, particularly females, setting and achieving a desirable body-fat level poses a problem. Many female runners set unrealistic targets—perhaps below their natural body-fat levels. This can result in a cycle of frustration and problems. Remember that the female body is designed to carry a higher level of fat than a male.

In studies, many female runners report eating a surprisingly low intake of kilojoules—less than you would expect for the training they do. It's not that they don't enjoy eating, in fact, many spend hours each day thinking about food. Rather, to keep body-fat levels down to what they consider to be suitable levels, these runners have to restrict energy intake. Often the situation becomes progressively worse—the more energy they restrict, the less they need to eat. It's almost as if the body is fighting to defend a higher body-fat level.

Some runners complicate the situation further by adding weird and wonderful diets, excessive training, and eating behaviour problems to their weight-loss techniques. Not all runners who practise anorexic (food restriction) or bulimic (bingeing) behaviours have a true eating disorder—many are driven to these actions in a desperate attempt to get on top of their body-fat goals.

If you are stressed or feel out of control with eating and your body fat, then your body-fat goals may not be right for you. The penalties associated with chasing unrealistic goals are twofold—the problems associated with how you get there, and then the problems faced by your body from literally being starved or overloaded. In the latter case, this might include disrupted periods and recurrent bouts of injury, illness or fatigue.

Read Chapters 1 and 2 to convince yourself that the key elements to a healthy diet are variety and an adequate kilojoule budget. If loss of body fat is a healthy option, then Chapter 3 will help you with a sensible plan of attack. If you seem caught up in a cycle of frustration, a sports dietitian, perhaps together with a sports psychologist, can help you to break free. You may have to settle for a slightly larger skinfold sum, but with your health and happiness improved, you will perform better in the long run.

### Amenorrhea, low bone density and stress fractures

It appears that female runners are more likely to suffer interruptions to their menstrual cycles—called secondary amenorrhea—than other athletes such as cyclists or swimmers. This is no longer regarded as a curiosity or a side-effect of training. Read Chapter 2.6, and the case history of Sharon below. Studies show that low estrogen levels in amenorrheic athletes can lead to loss of bone density—and bone strength and may increase the risk of stress fractures.

The picture is quite complicated, with many factors to consider. However the bottom line is that you should see a sports medicine doctor if your menstrual patterns become disrupted.

## Iron deficiency

Distance runners, particularly females, are at a high risk of low-iron status—perhaps even developing into iron deficiency anemia. As discussed in Chapter 2.5, many iron deficient athletes report feeling tired in training, but it is not until anemia has developed that performance is clearly impaired. Experts still argue about the severity of iron losses from gastrointestinal bleeding, sweat and red blood cell damage, but it is probable that the iron requirements of a runner will be increased. On paper, many runners look like they eat adequate dietary iron but on closer examination, this may be mostly non-heme iron, from plant food sources and it may not be well-absorbed.

Don, below, provides a typical story of a runner who overlooks his iron needs by focusing on carbohydrate intake only. For women runners the risk of iron deficiency is even greater, since their iron needs are increased (to cover menstrual blood loss), but their kilojoule budget is smaller. The iron story is covered below and in Chapter 2.5.

## Gastrointestinal problems

Many runners report gastrointestinal problems during hard runs, particularly races. It's hard to do a PB when you are suffering stomach cramps, diarrhea or wind. Some runners experience problems at the top end, with burping and heartburn, and a few even find that they pass blood during races.

The cause of these problems is unknown, but it seems to be related to the intensity of the running, the stress of competition and perhaps, dehydration. Some runners are able to pinpoint certain foods that cause problems, but this is an individual matter. Probably the best general advice is to experiment yourself with the type and timing of food that you consume before running. Often, it is best to run on an 'empty stomach', with pre-race or pre-training meals eaten well in advance. Liquid meal supplements such as Exceed Sports Nutrition Supplement or Sustagen make a good low-bulk, pre-exercise meal.

If problems persist, for important races you might need to literally achieve an empty gut, by switching to low-fibre foods and/or replacing meals with liquid meal supplements over the last 24 hours.

### Alternative dietary lifestyles

When many people take up running, they decide to make some dietary changes as well. Often it is all part of a healthy lifestyle change, but for some there is a belief in better performance with a better diet. It is great to see runners inspired to improve their eating patterns.

Some runners want to sweep through with a new broom, and embark on special dietary programs. Vegetarian diets and Pritikin diets are the most popular, and often claim to have the blessing of well-known runners. Both these dietary patterns have plenty to offer in terms of health and performance since both are based on the idea of increasing carbohydrate and fibre intake, and decreasing fat intake. However, they also have the potential to become very restricted and lacking in variety, particularly in the hands of highly motivated runners. Many runners make the mistake of concentrating on what should be given up rather than on preserving nutritional variety, moderation and flexibility.

Read the comments in Chapter 1 about how dietary changes can be made without sacrificing variety. By all means experiment with these diets, but from many points of view a better approach is to settle for a modified Pritikin or vegetarian diet, picking out the best bits and incorporating them into your own dietary patterns.

### Race preparation

The most critical dietary concern is to store sufficient muscle fuel to see out the event. A trained runner should not experience too much difficulty in preparing for events up to the 1/2 marathon. In Chapter 4.2 you will read that adequate muscle glycogen levels can be stored with a high-carbohydrate diet (daily intake of 9–10g per kg of body weight) and 24–36 hours of taper or rest. For weekly events, you may like to reschedule training sessions to achieve an adequate taper at the end of the week.

Carbohydrate loading is almost synonomous with the marathon—and rightly so. Races of this length and further will use up as much muscle glycogen as you can store. But despite the hype—or perhaps because of it—many runners do not know how to carbohydrate load properly. In the study reported below, some runners did a better job of 'garbo-loading' than 'carbo-loading'. Read Chapter 4.3 for the low-down on loading.

Runners who like to race with a light stomach can modify the fibre and bulk in their diets over the 12–24 hours before the event to reduce their gastrointestinal contents.

### The pre-event meal

With early morning races, it is tempting to sleep in for as long as possible—thus skipping breakfast. Other runners worry about gastrointestinal upsets if they eat a big breakfast before a race. However, the pre-event meal should not be sacrificed. It is the last opportunity to top up glycogen stores—particularly liver stores—and to top up fluid levels.

In many cases, a light snack, even a couple of pieces of toast and a drink, might be the best menu. If your race starts later in the day there might be time for a larger meal three to four hours pre-race. Don't forget fluids, especially if the day is hot, and pass up the last-minute sugar binge that you thought might provide quick energy. Your muscles should already be action-packed.

## Race fluids and fuel

For events up to the half-marathon, you should have all your fuel needs on board. Race nutrition should only need to be concerned with the prevention of severe dehydration. In races of this distance, the major threat of overheating comes from the pace at which you are running—the faster you run, the more metabolic heat you produce. But severe dehydration will add to the problem. So know your sweat losses and replace fluids to keep in touch with this.

In races of less than 10–15km in cool conditions, there may not be any need to drink during the event, and the top runners will not want to sacrifice any time. As the distance increases and/or the temperature rises, however, you will start to find aid stations along the route. Make use of these according to your sweat losses. If you are running for more than an hour, you should aim for a comfortable fluid intake —perhaps, 500–600ml spread over the race. Water is the most likely drink to be supplied, but a sports drink will also do the job.

For the marathon and above, performance will be enhanced by taking in carbohydrate during the run. This will be crucial for events of 50 miles or more. As explained in Chapter 4.7, an intake of about 50g of carbohydrate per hour is needed in events that go beyond the capacity of your muscle glycogen stores.

For most runners, replacing about 80 per cent of sweat losses will mean a fluid intake of 500–700ml/hr. With a sports drink of 7–8 per cent carbohydrate concentration, and an intake of about 200–250ml at each five kilometre aid station, fluid and carbohydrate needs are generally taken care of (you may need more on a very hot day). The front runners may have difficulty swallowing this amount, but in the middle of the pack you should be able to spare a little more time at the aid station.

In ultradistance races, 50 miles and more, runners even manage some solid food—but then they are often running at a relatively slower pace. Even so, most runners are best served by fluid forms of carbohydrate.

131

PROFILE: SHARON
*The bare bones of running*

Sharon couldn't believe her bad luck as she viewed the results of the CAT scan. The doctor pointed out the 'hot spot' in her lower leg—her second stress fracture that year. All that hard work and dedication down the drain.

The doctor agreed that it was unfortunate, but suggested that factors other than luck could be involved. He questioned Sharon about her training program and her diet, and listened as she described the lifestyle of a committed long distance runner.

Her training mileage fluctuated between 120 and 130km per week, mixed between track sessions and road running. Eighteen months ago she had had her first taste of international competition, and had come back from Europe with the view that the top women runners were all incredibly lean. Her project since then had been to minimise her body fat, and she worked diligently at this. While it was a constant struggle and required her to eat a sparrow-like and rigid diet, there was now little 'dead weight' on her body.

When the doctor asked Sharon if she had regular menstrual periods, she laughed.

'Of course not!' she said. 'Hardly any of the girls do. It's one of the rewards of all the hard work. In fact, often when we line up for a race, we ask around to see who's still having periods, and then you can feel happy that you've trained harder than them.'

The doctor explained to Sharon that amenorrhea in athletes was no longer considered harmless or a reward. As with menopause in older women, the loss of periods is associated with a drop in blood estrogen levels—and he reminded her that an important function of this hormone was to maintain bone mass. Studies have shown that amenorrheic athletes have lower bone density at some bone sites than normally menstruating athletes—and a higher incidence of stress fractures.

While it is tempting to conclude that amenorrhea leads to low bone density leads to stress fractures, the situation is more complicated. Stress fractures result from the failure of a bone to adapt to excessive trauma, and can occur whether bone density is low or normal, though a weakened bone is theoretically more likely to give way.

The doctor organised to sit down with Sharon and her coach and discuss the potential causes of an excessive training load—too much too quickly, hard surfaces, inadequate shoes and poor running style. Next on the agenda was to check her menstrual function and hormone levels, in case some non-sporting factor had caused her periods to stop just over a year ago. Being female, Caucasian and lightly framed was a risk factor for low bone density in itself, so a special bone scan was scheduled to measure her bone density against standards for a female of her age.

The main thrust of therapy to halt bone loss, and perhaps even restore levels, would be to restore low estrogen levels. The ideal situation, of course, would be for Sharon to resume a regular menstrual cycle—but this presumes we know why it happens in the first place. A number of factors have been blamed—low body fat, sudden loss of weight, eating disorders, intense training, and even the type of sport.

However, studies have failed to pinpoint a single or consistent culprit right across the board. Take the low body-fat theory, for example. Studies comparing groups of amenorrheic and normally-menstruating athletes have found no significant differences in the body-fat levels of each group. There were menstruating athletes with low body-fat levels and amenorrheic athletes with relatively high body-fat levels. It appears that individuals may have their own level of susceptibility to certain factors, and that a combination of factors may multiply the risk.

Some athletes can identify from experience the stress factors that seemed to push their bodies over the edge. For Sharon, trying to achieve an unnatural body-fat level for her was a possible factor. Before resorting to estrogen replacement treatment, the doctor decided it was worth trying to sort out Sharon's menstrual problems from within. He also suspected that her diet was inadequate in a number of respects other than a low kilojoule level, and explained that although a low calcium level, in itself, was unlikely to harm bone density, in the presence of low estrogen levels it might worsen the problem.

Sharon agreed to see a sports dietitian, who assessed the rigid dietary plan that she had followed over the past months (see table below). A nutrient analysis revealed that this diet was low in kilojoules compared to her estimated energy needs, and low in protein, carbohydrate, iron and calcium. Her typical daily calcium intake of about 300mg was below the Australian RDI of 800mg/day, and well below the 1000mg recommended for post-menopausal (and presumably other low-estrogen) women.

Sharon asked if she could remedy the situation with a calcium supplement. She had heard of other runners doing this to prevent stress fractures. The dietitian reminded her that the real problem was the amenorrhea, and advised that her diet needed total remodelling rather than a 'band-aid' approach.

To cut a long story short, Sharon's bone density was on the low side of the normal range. Nine months later it had improved a little. While reluctant at first to give up her low body-fat goals, she gradually conceded that the situation wasn't working and allowed herself to expand her dietary intake. The dietitian negotiated a daily plan of about 8400 kj per day (2000 Cals), which allowed her greater enjoyment and freedom with food, as well as greater nutrient intake. Even

**Sharon's diet before and after counselling**

|  | Before | After |
|---|---|---|
| Breakfast | Bowl of fruit salad (2 cups) 1 toast + Vegemite Black tea | Bowl of wholemeal cereal 200ml skim milk 1 toast + Vegemite 200ml orange juice |
| Lunch | Plain salad roll  Apple | Salad roll with reduced fat cheese, or slice of salmon (+ bones) Piece of fruit |
| Afternoon tea | Orange packet of sultanas | Carton of non-fat fruit yoghurt |
| Tea | 120g lean meat/chicken Medium potato  Small salad Low-joule jelly + Tbsp low-joule icecream | 120g lean meat/chicken Large potato or cup of rice/pasta 3–5 vegetables or salad Fruit salad + 100g low fat yoghurt/icecream |
| Supper | Slice of toast + vegemite | Milo or coffee made with skim milk In summer, iced milk drink |
| Analysis: Energy CHO Protein Calcium | 5200 kJ (1240 Cals) 200g 60g 310mg | 8400 kJ (2000 Cals) 350g 100g 1300mg |

though her body weight increased by 3kg, and her skinfold sum increased by nearly 10mm to 49mm, she agreed that she felt more energetic and less uptight at this level. Her periods resumed after four months probably due to changes in diet, training and stress.

With careful dietary choices she was able to achieve a calcium intake of 1000mg/day, eating low-fat, high-calcium foods such as skim milk, low-fat yoghurt and fish with bones. (See table above and Chapter 2.6 for more ideas). Many of the calcium foods could be turned into high-carbohydrate meals, thus meeting other training nutrition goals.

Sharon's running career has had no further hiccups to date. Her revised training program now includes less total mileage and some ongoing water running sessions—she became expert at this while the stress fractures healed. And she frequently lectures her running friends about seeing a sports doctor at the first sign of disruption to their periods.

PROFILE: DON
*Feeling ironed out?*

Don hadn't been training well for the last month. He felt tired all the time, despite plenty of sleep, and didn't feel as if he was recovering between training sessions. A 'run for fitness' man, he had decided six months ago to try a marathon, and had been doing things by the book in gradually stepping up his program. Strangely, he had coped better with the greater mileage at the beginning, and by now he had expected to be right on top of it. His knees niggled a bit, but one of his training partners kept him well-supplied with anti-inflammatory drugs and these seemed to keep it under control. He decided that perhaps he wasn't getting enough carbos, and decided to see a sports dietitian.

The dietitian questioned him about his symptoms, his training and his diet. Don described his daily meal routine, pointing out that he had put it together himself from a running magazine article. Not being a terrific cook, he had kept things simple—this included eating either rice or pasta each night.

The dietitian questioned him further about specific foods, and found that he didn't often eat meat (he believed it was too fatty for a runner). The same went for fish and chicken, though he sometimes ordered fish when eating at a restaurant. He didn't eat packaged breakfast cereals, but made his own muesli from rolled oats. As for legumes, silverbeet and spinach, he rarely ventured outside the conventional vegetables his mother had cooked for him at home. Dried fruit? A little in his muesli. Eggs? Too high in cholesterol. Vitamin or mineral supplements were not taken.

The dietitian suggested that iron deficiency, rather than carbohydrate deficiency, might be at the root of his fatigue problem. He was eating plenty of wholegrain bread, rice, pasta and oats for carbohydrate—and this was also his major source of dietary iron. Although his estimated iron intake appeared to be well above the Australian RDI for a male (7mg/day), almost all of his dietary iron was in the form least likely to be absorbed, i.e. non-heme iron. Nor did his meal mixtures make best use of factors to enhance iron absorption.

Additionally, it was likely that Don's iron requirements were increased above the general male RDI level. The increased training mileage, all run on hard surfaces wearing his favourite well-worn shoes, could be causing additional damage to red blood cells. And it was probable that the chronic use of anti-inflammatory drugs was causing a small but consistent loss of blood through gastrointestinal bleeding.

The dietitian organised for Don to see a sports doctor to discuss training and the appropriate use of anti-inflammatory drugs, and to order a blood test to determine his iron status. The results came back a few days later, the hemoglobin level normal, but at the low end of the range, and the ferritin level (a storage form of iron) quite low at 12ng/ml. While these tests are often hard to interpret (what is the best level for an athlete to have?), it seemed likely that Don was in the first stages of iron deficiency.

Experts disagree about the level at which iron deficiency actually affects performance, and it is probable that an athlete would have to become anemic (low hemoglobin level) before a measurable drop in performance could be detected. Nevertheless, many athletes report tiredness in training in the early stages—and the situation deserves treatment, if only to prevent it from continuing into severe iron deficiency.

The doctor and dietitian agreed on a program of high-dose iron supplements for six weeks, to boost iron stores while Don re-organised his dietary intake. Once his iron stores were topped up, Don would support his iron needs with iron from his food. The dietitian outlined the following nutrition plan for Don to follow:

- Continue with high-carbohydrate foods at each meal, but add a small portion of lean red meat, chicken, liver pate or shellfish to the menu. The principle of a low fat intake could be preserved.

- Add some iron-fortified breadfast cereal, such as Bran Flakes or Weetbix, to his muesli mix.

- Expand food choices by trying legumes, green leafy vegetables, and low-fat egg dishes.

- Add some vitamin C foods, such as orange juice, to any meal in which non-heme iron was the prominent source of iron.

She provided Don with some recipes and he began to experiment with cooking. While adding oysters and prawns to his stir-fried rice may sound exotic, there were some simple changes he could make also, such as ordering a roast beef and salad sandwich at lunch (saves him cooking a whole roast for one person.)

At the end of six weeks, Don reported feeling more energetic and more adept in the kitchen. His ferritin levels had increased to greater than 50ng/ml, so it was agreed to stop the supplement and retest in another six months. Pleased with this success, Don asked if it was all right for his training partners to take iron supplements if they also felt tired.

The dietitian agreed that many runners considered iron supplements a quick 'pick-me-up' for fatigue or else supplemented 'just in case of a deficiency'.

It was true that iron supplements could be bought over the counter of pharmacies. However, the dietitian pointed out that self-prescription and casual use of these supplements often led to an unnecessarily high intake of iron, with the potential for harm including interference with the absorption other body minerals such as zinc.

However, the real fault lay in seeking a simple solution for a complex problem. For a start, fatigue could be caused by a number of factors—including lack of sleep, overtraining and inadequate carbohydrate intake. These factors would not be rectified with an iron supplement.

Don was reminded that his own iron problem had been carefully assessed and comprehensively treated. His friends who self-diagnosed and self-treated would miss out on such expert advice. They might never discover or treat the underlying causes of the iron deficiency, nor benefit from counselling on all aspects of training nutrition. For example, there could easily be a medical condition causing the iron loss, such as an ulcer. Self-diagnosis and treatment could mean missing the chance for an early diagnosis.

Don went back to his squad with renewed vigour and steadily continued his marathon training program. At the last report, he was confidently counting the days until the big event.

*Carbohydrate loading—a load of?*

Picture the scene. You have been training hard for six months for the marathon, and there are only three days until the gun sounds. Now for the real fun. Good-bye Pritikin for the next couple of days while you create new records in pizza and chocolate eating. On the final evening, you organise a carbo-loading function with your training buddies, and fill your stomach to within an inch of bursting. Looking at the chocolate mousse, you wish you hadn't eaten so much lasagne. However, you find room on the way home for a couple of donuts convincing yourself that this will come in handy over the last ten kilometres. This carbohydrate loading is great stuff, right?

Wrong. Runners who practise this version of carbo-loading risk a double disservice—an uncomfortably full stomach and a questionable intake of carbohydrate for muscle glycogen storage.

In a study of the carbohydrate-loading techniques used by 76 runners competing in the 1983 Nike marathon in Canberra, the runners were questioned about their training and dietary program over the final week before the race. The results showed a variety of practices, with some depleting in the early part of the week, some tapering their training over the last three days and others continuing to do their normal training right up to race day. Chapter 4.3 explains the modified loading technique that is now recommended.

Of most interest were the high-carbohydrate diets eaten over the last three days before the event. A summary of the results shows the average intake per day:

**Dictary intake of runners carbo-loading for a marathon**

| | Mean | Range |
|---|---|---|
| Carbohydrate intake | 470g/day | 188g–960g |
| Energy intake | 14 600 kJ/day | 5800–28 400 kJ |
| Proportion of energy as carbohydrate | 53% | 31–83% |

For maximum muscle glycogen synthesis, a daily intake of 9–10g of carbohydrate per kilogram of your bodyweight has been recommended (see Chapter 4.3). For these runners, this would translate into approximately 600–700g of carbohydrate per day, taking up at least 60 per cent of total energy intake. Some of the runners in the group achieved these levels, but at the other end of the scale some managed only 200g or so of carbohydrate per day.

From the proportion of energy that came from carbohydrate in these loading diets, it is obvious that some runners did not understand carbohydrate foods and high-carbohydrate meals. With only 30 per cent of their total energy intake coming from carbohydrates, a few runners managed to eat *less* carbohydrate than would be found in the typical Australian diet—and in Chapter 1 we found that the typical food patterns in this country were already inadequate in carbohydrate intake.

So where did these runners go wrong? Read the hints for carbohydrate-loading in Chapter 4.3. The meal patterns described by the runners in the study showed the following classic mistakes:

- The runners continued to eat large amounts of non-carbohydrate foods at the meal, such as protein foods, and low-carbohydrate salads. Although these are part of a nutritious diet, the main goal of carbohydrate-loading days is to meet carbohydrate intake goals. You can afford to sacrifice some of these other nutrients to make more room on your plate and in your stomach for the carbos.

- The runners fell for the idea that 'junk foods' are good carbohydrate foods. A lot of them ate large amounts of foods they considered to be low in nutritional value—take-aways, chocolate, creamcakes and rich desserts. Most of these foods contributed more fat than carbohydrate to the diet.

- While many foods were correctly identified as high in carbohydrate, when made into a meal, the dish often had only a small amount of this important ingredient. A good example is lasagne: there would be few runners who haven't heard that pasta is a good carbo food, but many forget that lasagne recipes may contain only a few small sheets of pasta, and a lot of meat, oil and cheese. See table below for ways to replace high-fat carbo meals with the real thing.

- The runners continued their healthy habits of eating 'no added sugar' and artificially sweetened foods. While these food items might assist with keeping to a moderate sugar intake in the everyday diet, during the three days of carbo-loading before an event, it is okay to stray outside the usual dietary concerns. Canned fruit with added sugar and sweetened soft drinks are easy and compact ways to boost carbohydrate intake.

# IDEAS FOR REPLACING HIGH-FAT CARBOHYDRATE FOODS WITH A LOWER-FAT AND HIGHER-CARBOHYDRATE ALTERNATIVE

| High-fat carbo food | Alternative |
| --- | --- |
| Lasagne | Pasta—large serve with a small amount of low-fat meat or tomato sauce |
| Pasta with rich, creamy sauce (very filling) | Pasta as above |
| Crumpet soaking with margarine | Crumpet with honey or jam |
| Pancake soaking with whipped butter and/or cream | Pancake with honey or syrup— perhaps a little low-fat icecream |
| Croissant | Bagel or bread roll |
| Pizza with the lot | Thick crust pizza—vegetarian or seafood, with less cheese *OR* Make your own pizza—muffin or pita bread base, low fat toppings |
| French fries | Baked potato with low-fat filling |
| Donut | Coffee scroll (scrape of marg.) |
| Cream cake or pastry | Muffin or fruit loaf |
| Toasted muesli | Untoasted muesli and other breakfast cereals |
| Toasted ham/cheese sandwich | Toasted banana or baked bean sandwich—thick sliced bread and scrape of marg. |
| Thickshake | Fruit smoothie—skim milk, fruit low fat icecream/yoghurt |
| Chocolate bar | Plain muesli bars—especially low-fat brands |
| Chocolates/toffees | Jelly beans and jubes |

In this study, the group of runners who finished the marathon in less than three hours reported significantly greater training mileage and achieved a higher percentage of carbohydrate in their loading diets, than the runners who took more than 3.5 hours. This is of course only an observation and cannot prove directly that the extra carbos improved performance. It is just as likely that the good runners knew more about what they were doing, than that a good loading diet improved race times.

The moral of the story is that carbohydrate loading might be on the tip of every runner's tongue, but to get it right you need to carefully consider which foods go into your mouth.

See also the Profiles in Middle Distance Running for an account of Pritikin eating and gastrointestinal problems during running.

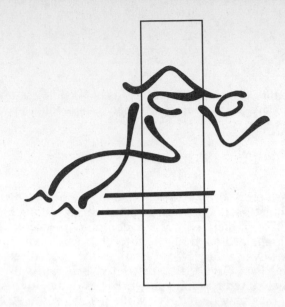

# Middle distance running

In this chapter running events ranging from 800 to 5000 meters are covered, with the common link being that each is run as a track race, and each requires the development of both aerobic and anaerobic energy supply systems.

Competition begins with school athletics, and continues through from club level to the international scene. In addition to World Championships and the Olympic Games, an international Grand Prix circuit of track and field meets is held each year, with a selected program of events rotating each season.

## Training

Middle-distance runners often train similarly to their long-distance counterparts in the off-season (traditionally winter) although total weekly mileage and the distance of their 'long runs' may be slightly less. Training is undertaken twice a day, with a mixture of continuous runs and track interval work. Some runners include weight training when time and facilities permit.

As the competition season approaches, greater emphasis is placed on track work and improvements in speed. There may be a drop in mileage as the quality of the sessions increases. Training is normally reduced over the days leading up to the race, depending on the importance of the event.

## Competition

Middle distance athletes normally specialise in one or two distances, such as the combination of 800m and 1500m races. At national and international level, an athlete will rarely compete in more than two races on the program, although at the interclub level some athletes will try themselves over a variety of distances. At specialised meets, such as the Grand Prix circuit, the restricted program will usually offer only one event suited to each runner. For example, in this year's program a 1500m race may be offered, while last year, the 800m race was featured.

The competitive season is traditionally summer. Athletes wishing to compete overseas, particularly in the opposite hemisphere, may have to organise their training to extend their competition peak, or to peak out of time to their own domestic scene. Interclub meets are held over a day, usually in the afternoon, with some athletes competing in a couple of different races. Some national and international track meets are held over a number of days, often with heats and semi-finals (if needed) on the same day, and the final on the following day. Events at such meets are generally held in the afternoon or evenings, although heats may be scheduled for mornings. Other European and Grand Prix meets involve a single evening's program of selected events, with a straight final between invited runners.

Middle distance events are not long enough to challenge the normal glycogen stores of a well-trained athlete. However, with athletes competing up to 15 to 20 times over a season, especially on the European and Grand Prix circuits where mid-week competitions can entice runners to compete three times in a fortnight, recovery of glycogen stores between races becomes an important issue. In general, the limiting factors during middle distance events result from the build-up of the products of anaerobic metabolism—lactic acid and hydrogen ions.

## Physical characteristics

The physical characteristics of a middle distance runner are quite similar to the long distance runner. Perhaps because middle distance runners are not required to transport their body weight so far, there is less penalty from being slightly heavier—particularly in terms of height or muscularity. However, body-fat levels continue to be low.

**Typical physique (elite middle-distance runners)**

|  | Male | Female |
|---|---|---|
| Height | 176–186cm | 168–172cm |
| Weight | 66–74kg | 52–64kg |
| Skinfolds | 34–42mm | 43–81mm |

## Common nutrition issues

Many of the nutritional issues of middle distance running are similar to those of long distance running, and only the differences will be discussed in this chapter. From the Distance Running chapter read the first seven points which cover shared features of the training diet. Case histories are provided below to explore Pritikin eating, and gastrointestinal upsets during running—common concerns in both sports.

The following competition nutrition issues are important to the middle distance runner.

### Race preparation

Middle distance runners do not need to carbohydrate-load for competition, since their normal glycogen stores will be more than adequate to see them through the event. With 24–36 hours of a high carbohydrate diet combined with rest or tapered training, a runner should be well-prepared for a race. Since races can be run at various times of the day, pre-race plans will vary. A breakfast or brunch-type meal will be suitable for events early in the day. If you are running in an evening race you might like to continue your normal meal plans until lunch and then finish with a light pre-race meal. Read Chapter 4 for more details.

### Post-race recovery

Hard running causes muscle fibre damage, and impairs the refilling of glycogen stores. Muscle glycogen storage is aided by providing a rapid supply of carbohydrate to the muscle. The first few hours are an important recovery period for a depleted muscle, and a damaged muscle will also make better use of carbohydrate during the first six hours than over the next 24–48 hours.

Make use of this window of opportunity to maximise your recovery, especially if you have a busy race calendar. Don't presume that race organisers will look after your needs. Bring your own supplies of fluid and carbohydrate—see Chapter 5 for ideas.

### Travelling on the circuit

For those lucky enough to compete on an international circuit, particularly the Grand Prix or European circuit, there are many challenges.

Some of these relate to being a travelling athlete, such as living out of suitcases and eating at restaurants. Another challenge comes from the compact competition schedule, which can mean ten big races in as many weeks. This timetable requires a quick recovery and preparation between events, over and over again. Juggling training and racing, not to mention transport schedules, accommodation details and money, can be exhausting. It is often hard to hold your peak—both physically and mentally.

The travelling athlete needs to plan well in advance, and to be aggressive about meeting nutritional goals on the road. An efficient preparation and recovery plan requires careful attention to finding the local carbohydrate foods, and clever scheduling of training between events. Look after immediate post-race recovery by consuming fluid and carbohydrate straight away. Again it may be wise to have your own recovery food supply—don't rely on the post-race party or a late-night meal in a foreign town. Get recovery on the road, and then take part in post-race celebrations—sensibly of course!

## PROFILE: STEVE
*Runner's trots*

At the finish of his last 5000m race, Steve doubled over with stomach cramps. It happened quite often in big events—pain, wind and the threat of diarrhea. Frequent pit-stops used to interrupt evening training, but he had gradually learned to control this by cutting out any afternoon snacks. However, the competition situation was still out of hand, and he feared that he might become another statistic in his running club—those who had to respond to an urgent 'call of nature' during a race.

His doctor organised a series of tests of his gastrointestinal function and reported that there were no obvious abnormalities. He suggested that an anti-diarrheal drug might help out in important events, but also that a session with the clinic's sports dietitian might result in a more comprehensive solution.

The dietitian placed the following checklist in front of Steve and invited him to look back over his experiences, searching for any common threads.

Steve considered this list carefully. There was no doubt that nerves played a role—he was often agitated before important races and could almost feel his stomach tie itself up in knots. He also remembered how anxious he had been before hard track sessions in his early days at the running club. There were plenty of problems in those days—just like last year around tax time when work had been incredibly busy and stressful. It didn't seem to matter how fast he ran, but how much he worried about how fast he ran.

Looking further down the list, Steve discounted the contribution of

## FACTORS POSSIBLY ASSOCIATED WITH RUNNER'S DIARRHEA

- Stress and nerves: do your symptoms get worse when you are nervous or stressed?
- Intensity of running: are symptoms worse during intense running— e.g. racing and training at or above race pace?
- Dehyration: a recent study has reported that dehydration increases the incidence of gastrointestinal complaints. Could this be adding to your problem—especially if you are withholding fluids in the belief that it could be the cause of your distress?
- Intake during exercise: do you consume concentrated drinks or solid foods during exercise? Perhaps you should experiment with a different program of fluid and carbohydrate intake. Does your sports drink contain a significant amount of fructose?
- Timing of pre-exercise meal: have you experimented with changing the time of your last food intake before training or racing?
- Size of pre-exercise meal: have you experimented with changing the amount of food eaten in the pre-exercise meal?
- Type of food in pre-exercise meal: have you experimented with changing the foods in your pre-exercise meal?
- Foods in your everyday diet: have you identified whether certain foods, or large quantities of certain foods, cause gut problems that become worse when you run?

  Examples:  too much fibre

  too much lactose (milk, icecream and milk-based products)

  too much fructose (fruits, some sports drinks)

dehydration to his problems, explaining that he was careful to keep his fluid levels topped up. Intake during exercise was also not relevant to Steve as a middle distance runner. Changing the timing and amount of food eaten before exercise to minimise gastrointestinal contents helped to reduce the diarrhea to a certain extent, although this tactic seemed to be self-limiting. He couldn't give up eating all together and he worried about fuelling up before important races. As for specific foods that caused problems, Steve could remember a couple of bad experiences before races—one with a bowl of untoasted muesli and another with a generous intake of stone fruit straight from the orchard. He'd learnt that too much fruit and too many raw oats didn't agree with him, at least not on the day of a race.

Steve described his usual meal patterns—seemingly a varied and moderate food schedule. The dietitian enquired further about Steve's intake of milk and milk products, and decided that there did not seem to be any evidence of intolerance to lactose (the sugar in milk).

Thus it seemed no single food or dietary factor was at fault. Rather, Steve's nervous state made his gut more active or susceptible to upsets. From the dietary view the dietitian suggested that he trial a program of reducing gastric contents before less important races. It would be hard to simulate race stress in training, so Steve prepared to experiment with some of the early races in the competition calendar.

For the 24–36 hours pre-race he would eat only low-fibre foods, and on the day of the race he would consume only a liquid meal supplement. A low-lactose supplement was recommended, such as Exceed Sports Nutrition Supplement, to avoid any complications from a sudden increase in lactose intake. By race time—late afternoon—he should be feeling light and untroubled.

Steve tried this on a couple of occasions and reported an improvement, not just in his gut symptoms, but in his pre-race anxiety levels. Worry about his gut problem was indirectly adding to the problem. The thought that medication provided still another avenue was comforting, but for the moment Steve decided to leave this as as something to fall back on. In fact, a stress management course offered at work has since taken his fancy, and he has decided to work on relaxation techniques for pre-race as well as everyday stress relief.

## PROFILES: TOM, DICK AND HARRY
*Pritikin eating*

The late Dr Nathan Pritikin wrote a series of best-selling books in the early 1980s promoting his diet and exercise program, which claimed to reverse coronary heart disease, achieve weight loss, and improve vigour and mental acuity. For endurance athletes he promised improved performance, specifically covered in the 1985 book *Diet for Runners*. At a wider level, he caused a great number of people to rethink their eating habits, and to take greater responsibility for their health and performance. His work has produced off-shoots such as special Pritikin foods, Pritikin-style restaurants, recipe books and health resorts—all devoted to helping achieve a low-fat, low-salt, high complex-carbohydrate diet.

While these principles agree with the dietary guidelines for good health, not to mention the optimum training diet for an athlete, Pritikin preached a more extreme message than nutrition experts would have liked. He recommended that fat intake be kept below 10 per cent of total energy, with 10–15 per cent of energy coming from protein and 80 per cent from complex carbohydrates. In addition he advocated that people abstain from any alcohol, caffeine, sugar and added salt, and that vitamin supplements were unnecessary and even dangerous.

Pritikin's message and his writing are emotive—full of dramatic warnings about the health consequences of eating the American or Western diet, and full of inspiring testimonials from people whose lives were enhanced by following his program. And although his program requires quite dramatic and rigid changes to eating and lifestyle habits, self-discipline is a familiar and often-prized characteristic of many athletes.

While the principles of the Pritikin diet can be appraised, it is probably more relevant to appraise an individual's *interpretation* of the diet. There are as many versions of 'Pritikin eating' as there are Pritikin followers, and in many cases, what makes the diet helpful or harmful to an athlete, is how the individual has put theory into practice.

For example, let's say that a year ago, Tom, Dick and Harry joined an athletics club with the goal of racing middle distance in interclub competition. They had all been successful at school athletics, and looked forward not only to the health and fitness benefits from training, but to carving their niche in Master's level competition. They threw themselves into their sport, enthusiastically adopting the training, the equipment, the language and lifestyle of runners. Pritikin's *Diet for Runners* was purchased by each and taken home. Twelve months later, we check their progress.

Tom, a perfectionist, has followed the Pritikin book almost to the letter. The very day the book was purchased he cleaned out his fridge and pantry of all 'illegal' foods. Out went cheese, egg, toasted muesli, icecream, the salt shaker and his after-work beers. He liked the simplicity of the 'seven survival staples' and basically formed his diet around these foods—wholemeal rice, kidney beans, steamed chicken, tomato-vegie sauce, frozen bananas, stewed apples and berries, and cottage cheese 'mock cream'.

Tom's wife was sceptical at first but has now resigned herself to his regimented diet, even if she does call it a 'desert island menu' or 'army rations' behind his back. On the nights that he is late home from training, she lets him cook his own meals. However, on weekends when the family eats together, she pores through recipe books to come up with low-fat, low-sugar meals that they can all eat. Entertaining guests is quite difficult. She misses her gourmet cooking, and complains that Tom's coffee substitutes don't finish off the meal with the same flourish as a brew of freshly ground coffee. They no longer dine out as regularly. Their friends seem a bit reluctant to fiddle around with menus and restaurants to suit Tom or perhaps they have tired of his lectures on how they are poisoning themselves with their eating habits.

Strangely enough, Tom doesn't actually look the picture of health that he promotes. He is pale, gaunt and drawn, having lost seven kilos in the first two months of the diet. To prevent further weight loss he has had to ignore some of the food quotas on the Pritikin maintenance scheme, and increase his intake of fruit and low-fat dairy products. His running is progressing adequately, but he doesn't always feel as 'supercharged' as the book promised.

Dick began his diet as enthusiastically as Tom, and for the first six months matched him rice cake for rice cake. He lost weight, his running progressed and then with an air of complacency he began to lose interest in the dietary regimentation. Some aspects were easy to keep up. He had successfully banished red meat, eggs, dairy products other than skim milk, and most packaged foods from his menu.

But gradually he began to reintroduce some of the foods that he missed. Treats included margarine on his toast, a weekly meal of fish and chips or a well-known burger chain meal, and Homer Hudson Icecream (after all, it comes in a pretty small tub). Everything in moderation, he told himself, so an occasional chocolate nibble wouldn't upset the good work achieved by the rest of his diet. And at the bakery after Sunday's long run, he often slipped a few choc-iced donuts in with the Pritikin buns.

Dick hasn't noticed the creeping weight gain, nor has he connected the occasional fatigue in training with his diet. He still considers himself a Pritikin devotee, and ordered a Pritikin meal at the Club Christmas Dinner.

Harry also believes in moderation, but his interpretation is different to Dick's. He read the Pritikin book, followed by a couple of other books on sports nutrition and nutrition for health, and he noticed that many of Pritikin's ideas overlapped with the views of the dietitians and nutritional scientists. Instead of overturning his diet completely, he decided to work on gradual improvements using some of the Pritikin strategies as a guide.

He began by concentrating on lower-fat meals, replacing fatty meats and dairy products with trimmed and low-fat versions and experimenting with low fat cooking methods. He reduced the size of his protein serve, leaving room to explore the world of carbohydrate foods. His wife cooked some new dishes from Pritikin recipe books, and used the principles to successfully modify some of the family's favourite recipes as well. Rather than moving along a pathway of increased food restriction, Harry found that his diet was actually expanding.

Harry and his wife eat out regularly, finding that with careful selection from the menu, and occasionally special requests, they can enjoy a healthy meal. However, they often try Pritikin-style restaurants, looking for new ideas for family meals. The transition has been gradual and painless, though Harry can mark his success by his trim figure and his training vigour.

Harry's modified Pritikin diet has an energy spread of 65 per cent carbohydrate, 12 per cent protein and 23 per cent fat, with all nutrients exceeding the recommended dietary intakes. Harry achieves the best of all possible worlds—nutritional goals for training and health, food enjoyment, support from family and friends and a flexible outlook.

Tom's diet, on the other hand, is modelled strictly on the Pritikin principles—with an energy intake ratio of 80 per cent carbohydrate, 8 per cent fat and 12 per cent protein. However, he has trouble meeting total energy needs from his unchanging and bulky food choices, and sometimes even fails to eat enough carbohydrate. With such a limited food range, his diet may also be limited in minerals and other nutrients. He has had to sacrifice the social and enjoyment aspects of food, although he is still too enthusiastic (or obsessed) to notice it.

Interestingly, Dick's diet has the same energy distribution as Harry's diet—about 65 per cent carbohydrate and 25 per cent fat. However, his vitamin and mineral intake is much lower, and has the same potential inadequacies as Tom's. And unlike Harry, who used his extra fat intake to allow him to eat nutritious foods such as reduced-fat dairy products and red meats, and to increase his social flexibility, Dick's dietary lapses have been splurges on high-fat, lower-nutrient value foods. Since his diet is erratic, switching from high-fat days to rigid Pritikin days, he sometimes fails to meet his carbohydrate needs for training or racing. And his weight will generally follow an upward trend as he grows fonder of his treats.

Hopefully, Tom and Dick will update their reading with the new books from the Pritikin Foundation, written by Nathan's son, Robert. The message has moved towards greater moderation and flexibility—practices which are already part of Harry's world. The Pritikins do not have a monopoly on healthy eating for runners or any other athletes, and it is not necessary to follow their diet completely and faithfully. However, we do owe a debt to the Pritikin influence for helping to commercialise and popularise attention to the way we eat.

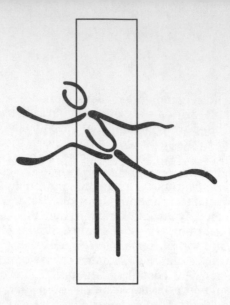

# Jumps, sprints and hurdles

Track and field competition includes a number of events of short duration that rely primarily on the development of power through anaerobic energy. At Olympic-level competition, sprint events include the 100m, 200m and 400m, as well as 4 × 100m and 4 × 400m relay events. Hurdle events are contested over 100m (women), 110m (men) and 400m. The jumps consist of the high jump, long jump, triple jump and pole vault.

Competition begins with school athletics, and an amateur athletics career can continue through club competition to international events—the most important being the Olympic Games, the World Championships and the expanding international Grand Prix circuit. While a full program of events is included at major competitions spanning a couple of days, at specialised meets such as Grand Prix competitions there is a selected program which rotates each year.

Sprint running also has a strong professional competition circuit, but in recent years we have seen a dismantling of the traditional barriers between amateur and professional running. A number of former professional runners have crossed to amateur competition to compete in state, national and even international competitions. Similarly, amateur athletes now compete in professional races with any prize money being paid into trust accounts.

## Training

The competitive season usually spans five to six months over the summer period. At the school and club level, many athletes will not train specifically during the off-season. Many are involved with other sports or study, and turn their attention to athletics only a month before the start of the interclub season. During the competition season they may train three or four evenings a week and compete on the weekend.

At the elite level, athletes train all year around with the base or off-season training involving around eleven sessions per week. Since an important component of success in these events is the ability to generate power relative to body weight, off-season training usually involves a considerable commitment to weight training, with about one-third of the total training load being carried in the gym.

The other emphasis of off-season training is the refinement of technique. In addition to running sessions on the track, drill sessions are conducted, for example, to improve leg speed or knee lift. As the competitive season approaches, track work increases to include more intervals and sprints, although technical work and weight training are still maintained.

The pre-competition taper does not need to be as severe as that practised by middle and long distance runners, since sprinters are already training for quality rather than quantity.

## Competition

Sprinters and jumpers can compete regularly at weekend or mid-week interclub meets during the season, but usually target three to six events in their calendar as being of greater importance. Athletes wishing to compete overseas must be ready for a an additional season, requiring them to work towards double or even triple peaks in their competition preparation.

At the interclub level, athletes often compete in a number of events conducted on the same day of a meet—for example a couple of sprints of different lengths, a jumping event and a relay race. At national and international level, athletes will only be qualified to compete in their major event and perhaps one relay, and events may be spread out over days of a meet. Depending on the size of the field there may be heats, semis and finals in the sprints and hurdles, and a qualifying round leading to the jump finals. The finals may be held on the same or next day to the qualifiers, depending on the length of the meet.

Even though the event itself involves a brief explosion of energy, a competition such as a jump may drag out for many hours while all competitors take their turn. The athlete's fuel stores are not a limiting factor in competition. Muscle ATP and creatine-phosphate systems are the most important energy source for events lasting seconds and are quickly regenerated between bouts. Anaerobic metabolism of carbohydrate plays a greater role during events lasting up to a minute, but muscle glycogen stores are not depleted by events of this duration.

## Physical characteristics

Sprinters and jumpers typically share the low body-fat levels of distance runners, since power-to-weight ratio is an important determinant of performance. Muscle mass is typically higher, accounting for some of the higher total body weight. However, these athletes also tend to be taller than distance runners particularly the jumpers.

**Typical physique (elite sprinters)**

|  | Male | Female |
| --- | --- | --- |
| Height | 172–185cm | 166–181cm |
| Weight | 67–81kg | 60–69kg |
| Skinfold sum | 32–52mm | 45–88mm |

**Typical physique (elite jumpers)**

|  | Male | Female |
| --- | --- | --- |
| Height | 178–190cm | 172–183cm |
| Weight | 67–83kg | 55–71kg |
| Skinfold sum | 41–73mm | 41–73mm |

## Common nutrition issues

### Low body-fat levels

Low body-fat levels usually occur naturally for male athletes, thanks to the cumulative effect of training on the right genetic stock. Some female sprinters and jumpers may have to manipulate their food intake and training to achieve their desired body-fat levels, but there is generally not the same desperation as seen amongst female distance runners. Club-level athletes of both sexes who reduce or cease training over the off-season may need to lose body fat at the beginning of the next competition season. Where help is needed in this regard, read Chapter 3 for sensible and successful methods.

### Training nutrition

The goals of training nutrition are discussed in Chapters 1 and 2. Matching carbohydrate intake to training needs is still a priority for sprint-type athletes, although understandably, carbohydrate requirements do not reach the levels of endurance-type athletes.

If you are unsure whether your eating plans meet your nutritional goals, a sports dietitian is the best person to assess your diet and guide you. Even if you think you are eating well, you may learn new ways to expand and enjoy your nutritional horizons—and getting a stamp of approval can be a great confidence boost. See Andrew's story below.

### Preparation for competition

Since jumps and sprints will not deplete muscle glycogen stores, carbohydrate loading before a competition provides no advantages. In fact the gain in body weight from additional glycogen and water is simply extra weight to carry, and is therefore a possible disadvantage to performance—especially in jumps and hurdles where you must lift yourself off the ground as well as propel yourself forward.

The day of competition is best tackled with glycogen stores topped up to their usual resting level. With a high-carbohydrate diet already in place for training needs, glycogen levels can be restored easily before competition with 24–36 hours of rest or very light training.

### Competition day food and fluid

The role of the pre-competition meal is discussed in Chapter 4.4. Choose a high-carbohydrate meal that suits the time of your event and your personal preferences. If you are competing early in the morning, for example in a heat, you may only have time for a light breakfast. Late afternoon and evening events may allow you to eat your everyday breakfast, and even lunch, finishing off with a small snack two to three hours before the event. Experiment in training if an important competition is coming up and you are programmed to compete at an unaccustomed time. Take care to drink plenty of fluids when you are competing in hot weather.

Although your sport technically lasts only seconds or minutes, competition may be a drawn-out affair. Your day can become a number of all-out efforts interspersed with variable amounts of waiting around in between. What should you eat and drink between events, or during events that sprawl out over hours?

Your nutritional goals are to keep hydrated, to maintain blood sugar levels and to feel comfortable—avoiding hunger but not risking the discomfort of a full stomach. How you will do this largely depends on the time interval between events or efforts. See Bernadette's account below for ideas, and like her, be organised to look after your own needs.


PROFILE: BERNADETTE
*A long day on the track*

Despite being the most promising sprinter in the region, at last year's interschool athletics carnival, Bernadette could only manage one bronze medal. Her program had been busy—heats of the 100m at 9.15, long jump at 12.30pm, final of the 100m at 3.00pm and the 4 × 100m relay at 4.15pm. The morning of the meet was rushed, hurrying to get across town to the sports ground of the host school. Bernadette had forced herself to swallow a mouthful of toast as she raced out the door. She consoled herself that she was too nervous to eat anyway.

By mid-morning, with the 100m heats out of the way, Bernadette was ravenous. She eagerly scoured the sports ground kiosk for something light to eat—after all, the long jump was not far off. The offerings were limited to pies, hot dogs, soft drinks and chocolate bars. She chose the chocolate 'for energy' and made her way to the jump pit. With so many competitors, the long jump stretched out for nearly two hours and as she sat out on the oval awaiting her next jump, Bernadette felt herself become hot and sunburnt. It was hard to concentrate and she jumped badly.

There was barely enough time to warm up for the 100m final, let alone get to the amenities block on the other side of the sports ground to find a tap. She ran, feeling tired from a dull headache. She finished the day with a third place in the relay event—small comfort for the hours of training she had completed over the past three months.

This year the story was quite different, although her training was unchanged and the meet program was almost the same as the previous year. The difference was a careful plan for competition day, organised in collaboration with the school's new athletics coach.

Bernadette rose earlier than usual to allow herself to have a light but relaxed breakfast of cereal and fruit juice before leaving for the sports ground. Not willing to rely on the ground catering, she brought with her a picnic basket of provisions for the day—foods that she had tested out in training over the previous month.

Once the 100m heats were over, Bernadette had a small meal of honey sandwiches and fruit juice, knowing that these would be comfortably digested before the jumps started in two hours' time. Once they called for competitors in this event, she set up a 'camp' on the oval near the jumps pit, bringing with her a drink bottle full of cold sports drink, and a small beach umbrella for shade. Some of the other competitors laughed at the sight but were soon feeling the heat of the midday sun and wishing they had done the same.

With a victory and a personal best in the long jump, Bernadette commenced her warm-up for the 100m final and followed up soon after with her second gold medal for the day. With just over an hour before the relay event there was little time to eat solid food. Feeling a little empty, Bernadette was glad she had a can of Exceed Sports Nutrition Supplement on ice in her picnic basket. Refreshed and re-vitalised, she prepared for the last event and helped her team win a silver medal.

While Bernadette knows that her medals were not just the result of particular food or drinks, her careful organisation did allow her to do justice to her talent and training, rather than see it wasted with careless race-day mistakes.

## PROFILE: ANDREW
*How does a dietitian assess a diet?*

Andrew, a 400m hurdler, is aiming for selection in next year's World Cup athletics team. He has been interested in sports nutrition for the last two years, gleaning information from his coach, from articles in Runner's World and from the occasional sports medicine seminar. He has tried to incorporate these ideas into his own diet, although he is not always sure which foods are involved.

Wanting to leave nothing to chance in his running career, Andrew decided to seek professional opinion on whether his diet was as good as he thought it was. He made an appointment to see the sports dietitian at the nearby sports medicine clinic, and his first question was: 'How will you tell if I'm eating well? Will you do a hair analysis or something?'

The dietitian explained that hair analysis, along with practices such as live-cell microscopy and iridology (eye examination), fall into 'alternative' medicine therapy and are not generally regarded as valid measures of nutritional status. The results are open to misinterpretation and do not fit in with the conventional scientific view of nutrition.

A dietitian's major assessment tools are body composition measurements (usually skinfolds), information on lifestyle and exercise patterns, and a careful assessment of food intake patterns. Medical information may be needed, including an examination for signs and symptoms of various nutritional conditions. Sometimes the dietitian will also require biochemical tests in order to confirm a suspicion of a nutritional problem.

Since biochemical tests are expensive and occasionally a nuisance to the subject, they are best undertaken only when the other information points to a possible problem. For example, it not necessary for athletes to have hundreds of tests to see if they are deficient in one or more of the vitamins or minerals. However, if symptoms of iron deficiency are apparent, and the athlete's usual eating patterns were assessed to fall short of their estimated iron requirements, then it would be useful to take the appropriate blood tests to confirm iron status.

Andrew's nutritional assessment began with a discussion about his sporting commitment—his goals, training and immediate competition plans. The dietitian then asked about his interest in nutrition and any special dietary ideas he was already following. Did he live at home with his family, in an institution, alone, or in a shared house? Who did the shopping and cooking? What else did he have to fit into his day apart from training—university, full-time work or part-time job?

The discussion turned to body weight and body fat, with Andrew explaining that his body weight never fluctuated more than one or two kilograms at any time of the season. He showed her the results of a recent body-fat check, taken by his coach according to the Australian Institute of Sport sum of skinfold procedure. His score for the sum of eight skinfold sites was 38mm—very lean.

Next, the dietitian took a dietary history from Andrew, asking him to recount a typical day's eating plan. She led him through the day, noting his activities—particularly training—and typical food habits. It was a gentle but thorough interrogation, drawing a detailed account of the types, timing and quantities of foods and drinks consumed, noting how it was cooked or prepared, and why it was chosen. Special attention was focused on intake before, during and after training.

Weekends were described separately, looking for any changes to usual weekday patterns. Separate questions looked at eating out, take-aways, and other changes to the routines just described, such as differences in summer and winter eating. Competition nutrition was then explored, looking at any special dietary preparation, pre-race meals and tactics for race-day food and fluids.

'What can you learn from this?' Andrew asked. The dietitian explained that, providing Andrew had been able to accurately describe his usual eating patterns, this profile could provide a good general assessment of his success in meeting his nutritional goals. Not only did it look at what was consumed, but it helped to explain some of the reasons why it was chosen. This was important to know, especially when improvements were advised. For example, knowing that food availability or finances stood in the way of a better food choice would call for different tactics than if lack of nutrition knowledge was the only problem.

To complete the picture, Andrew was invited to keep a food diary. The dietitian explained that this was like having a video made of a person's golf swing or swimming stroke. By recording food intake over a period of time, Andrew could step back and look at it objectively, comparing actual intake with what he thought he was eating, and with what he should be eating for optimal performance. With accurate descriptions of the quantity quantities eaten and drunk, a computerised dietary analysis could be undertaken, estimating daily intake of kilojoules and nutrients.

Of course, to do justice to the exercise, special skills must be applied both by the athlete and the dietitian. Andrew was instructed in the special tactics of keeping a good food record. Firstly, he needed to make sure that the period of recording reflected his usual eating patterns, and secondly he needed to learn techniques to accurately describe the type and amount of food and drink consumed. He then completed a diary for seven days using these skills, describing a full week of training and an interclub meet.

For her part, the dietitian utilised her special nutrition knowledge and training in using the computer dietary analysis program to estimate Andrew's daily nutrient intake. Although she scrutinised day-to-day variation in intake, most interest was focused on the average daily nutrient intake—a reflection of his typical diet. The results of this are presented in the table below along with a description of typical meal plans and the recommended dietary intakes set for Australians (RDIs).

To evaluate Andrew's diet, the dietitian worked through the checklist of goals of training and competition nutrition.

- Suitability of body weight and body fat: Andrew's daily kilojoule intake is appropriate, maintaining his body fat at a low level to suit his sport.

- Adequacy of nutrient intake: The intake of all nutrients included in the analysis is well in excess of the RDIs even where requirements may be increased by heavy exercise. This is partly due to Andrew's generous energy intake, but is also due to his careful choice of nutritious foods. His enjoyment of a wide food variety is an important asset.

- Recovery: Andrew has done well to make carbohydrate his principal energy source, thus supplying plenty of fuel to restock his muscles after each training session. Although his carbohydrate requirements do not reach the extreme levels of an endurance athlete, training twice a day still places a load on muscle glycogen stores. As well as looking after his total intake of carbohydrate, Andrew cleverly promotes recovery by timing a carbohydrate meal or snack to immediately follow each training session. Fluid replacement is also well looked after.

- Long-term nutrition issues: Andrew's diet meets the dietary guidelines for good health being moderate in fat and salt intake, and focused on a variety of nutritious carbohydrate and fibre foods. As well as looking after his immediate sporting goals, this diet should lessen his risk of nutrition-related diseases in later life.

- Competition nutrition. Andrew uses interclub meets to practise strategies that he will use in more important competition. He has fine-tuned his preparation and pre-race meal and takes his own food when he travels to an interstate meet. It is better to be safe than sorry!

The dietitian congratulated Andrew , assuring him that his diet met his nutritional goals as a hurdler. All that was left to make his diet

**A nutrient analysis of a typical day's eating for Andrew (hurdler, 78kg)**

Typical food patterns

Training

Breakfast: straight after training at home
Wholegrain cereal-e.g. Weetbix, Sustain, OatBran
large bowl (75g) + 300ml low-fat milk
2 sl. of wholemeal toast + scrape of marg + jam
250ml fruit juice
Plenty of water

During morning: water, particularly if warm day

Lunch: at work
2 wholemeal rolls with scrape of marg OR mayonnaise (never both)
low fat filling of chicken, salmon, egg or roast beef
Salad
Scone or muffin   unbuttered
250ml fruit juice
Piece of fruit

Training after work

On way home from training:   500ml fruit juice
2 plain muesli bars

Dinner: home, later in evening
Medium serve (120g) of lean meat, fish and chicken
Large serve of potatoes, rice, pasta or noodles
3–4 other vegetables
(all cooking low-fat)
Dessert: fruit or fruit salad with low-fat yoghurt or
low-fat icecream
Water

Average daily energy and nutrient intake

|  | Andrew's diet | RDI |
|---|---|---|
| Energy | 13 340 kJ | |
| | 3185 Cals | |
| Protein | 140g | |
| | = 1.8g/kg body weight | 1g/kg[a] |
| Carbohydrate | 540g | |
| | = 6.9g/kg | 6–8g/kg[a] |
| Fat | 79g | |
| Alcohol | — | |
| Vitamin A (retinol) | 2675µg | 750µg |
| Vitamin B1 | 3.5mg | |
| (thiamin) | = 0.26mg/1000 kJ | 0.10mg/1000 kJ |
| Vitamin B2 | 4.3mg | |
| (riboflavin) | = 0.32mg/1000 kJ | 0.15mg/1000 kJ |
| Vitamin B3 | 69mg | |
| (niacin equivalents) | =·5.2mg/1000 kJ | 1.6mg/1000 kJ |
| Vitamin C | 525mg | 40mg |
| Iron | 33mg | 7mg[a] |
| Calcium | 1120mg | 800mg |
| Zinc | 20mg | 12mg |

Energy contribution—general training

| | | |
|---|---|---|
| Carbohydrate | 60% | 50–60%[a] |
| Fat | 22% | 20–30% |
| Protein | 18% | 12–15% |

*Notes*:  [a] taken from Chapter 2—estimated requirements for a moderate training load
*Sources*:  Nutrient analysis: NUTTAB 1987; Australian Department of Community Services and Health
    RDIs: *Recommended Nutrient Intakes, Australia*, NHMRC, 1990.

ideal was confidence that he was eating well, and enjoyment of his food. Not only would such a diet meet his physiological needs but it would give him a psychological edge. In top competition, Andrew would be well served by these advantages.

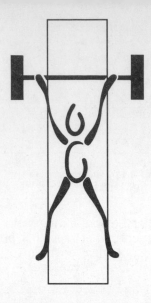

# Strength sports: Olympic weightlifting, powerlifting and throwing events

In lifting and throwing events, performance is based on the generation of explosive power for a couple of seconds, relying almost completely on anaerobic energy. Muscle ATP and creatine-phosphate are broken down to supply the energy for a single effort, and are quickly regenerated between bursts.

The throwing events include the javelin, shot put, discus and hammer. Athletes compete openly against each other in these field events. Weightlifting is also an Olympic event, with competitors being grouped into categories according to their bodyweight. There are ten bodyweight divisions ranging from flyweights (below 52kg) to the super heavyweights (over 110kg). Olympic weightlifters perform two lifts—

the snatch and the clean and jerk. The competition recognises both individual lifts as well the combined total.

Powerlifting is not an Olympic event. It uses the same body weight categories as the weightlifters, and judges the overall weight lifted during three lifts—the bench press, the squat and the dead lift. Although women compete in all lifting and throwing events, powerlifting and weightlifting are dominated by men.

## Training

At school or club level, athletes may not train all year round. However, as the level of competition increases, so does the training commitment, both in terms of a year-round program, and in terms of an increased number of training sessions per week. As with endurance sports, it is not possible to maintain a peak for prolonged periods of time, so training is organised into a series of cycles leading to a peak during the competition season, usually summer. Athletes competing internationally may have to peak for two or three competition seasons each year.

The training focus of power athletes varies with the skill demands of their event and the time of the season. Lifters concentrate on weight training, and in the case of Olympic weightlifting (which involves greater technique), flexibility. Throwers divide their training time between weight training, running and speed work, flexibility work and technique training.

In the off-season or in base training, the main focus is on increasing muscle bulk and strength through more general weight training. The number of sets and repetitions undertaken in a weight training session is larger at this time of the season, providing stimulus for muscle hypertrophy and strength gains.

As the competition season approaches, the repetitions are reduced and the poundage raised to increase power output. More time is spent fine-tuning the technique of events.

## Competition

The throwing events allow three throws per competitor, with the leading eight being given a further three throws to decide the placings. The competition is conducted without a break and may take one or two hours to complete. In large international competitions a qualifying round may be held on the day before the final, with a qualifying distance being set for entry into the final.

The lifting events allow each competitor three attempts at each lift category, with the competitor nominating the weight they wish to lift.

There is a break between each section of lifts. Weigh-in occurs about an hour before the commencement of the competition.

## Physical characteristics

Since strength is related to muscle mass, the typical thrower or lifter has a large body weight and muscle mass. In the throwing events, being non-weight matched, body-fat levels can also be high—even by community standards. Unless body-fat levels become so high that body shape interferes with technique or general health is at risk, there seems less penalty for throwers to carry extra body fat. The exception is javelin throwers who have a longer run-up prior to throwing, and who need to generate as much speed as possible over this distance. Javelin throwers would be expected to have the lowest body-fat levels amongst throwers.

Lifters, being classified into weight divisions, will show a great variety of body weights and body-fat levels. In the lower weight divisions, maximum strength will be achieved by maximising muscle mass and minimising body-fat levels. Thus a weightlifter in the fly and bantam weight divisions should strive for low body-fat levels. As the weight divisions increase, body-fat levels increase along with muscle mass, although it is not until heavy weight and super heavy weight divisions that lifters can be less concerned about their power to weight ratio.

## Common nutrition issues

*Bulking-up—how much protein do you need?*

In Chapter 3.6 the necessary ingredients for a successful bulking-up program were listed as:

* the right parents
* the right training load
* the right diet.

Hopefully the first two ingredients have been taken care of, and all that stands in the way of you and success is your diet. What constitutes the right diet is a point of difference between strength-training athletes and most sports scientists. The folklore in strength sports is that a high protein intake is required—up to 3g/kg of body weight, or up to 20 per cent of total energy intake, figures that are supported by Eastern bloc scientists.

However, as discussed in Chapter 2.3, the consensus of most sports scientists is that while the protein needs of strength-training athletes are increased, such high levels are not necessary. A figure of up to

1.5g of protein per kilogram of body mass is recommended during times of muscle growth, although adolescents may require 2g/kg during total body growth spurts. Dietary surveys of strength-training athletes generally report that these protein intake levels are easily reached. For example, the weightlifters studied below were estimated to consume nearly 160g of protein per day, supplying 1.8g/kg body weight.

Unfortunately, many strength athletes chasing protein foods end up eating high-fat diets. The diets of the weightlifters below, and diets of other strength athletes reported in studies, contain just on 40 per cent of energy from fat—which contributes neither to protein nor carbohydrate needs. Read Chapters 1 and 2 to reorganise your ideas about the optimum training diet. In particular, Chapter 2.3 lists protein foods that are low-fat or high-carbohydrate, suggesting ways to achieve all nutritional goals simultaneously.

The key issue for bulking up is really energy intake. A high energy intake from nutritious food will also be high in protein, carbohydrate, vitamins and minerals. The account of Paul below illustrates that some athletes still find difficulty in consuming sufficiently high energy intakes. Read how to overcome this by being organised, and planning frequent compact meals and high-energy drinks.

## Dietary supplements

Another area of folklore in strength sports is the need for dietary supplements, both to meet physiological nutrient needs and to provide direct ergogenic benefits. Many studies of strength athletes have reported heavy use of various dietary supplements. Read Chapter 6 and the account of the weightlifters below so that you can make up your own mind.

## Body fat—optimising power to weight ratios

Although in some lifting and throwing events, a high body-fat level is not a great disadvantage, there are some instances in which athletes could benefit by reducing their body-fat levels. The best example of this is in the low and middle weight divisions of weightlifting and powerlifting, where you will derive an advantage over your opponents by being at the greatest muscle mass (and therefore lowest body-fat level) that is possible for your weight limit—a higher power to weight ratio.

Many lifters do not seem to appreciate this. It is almost a universal practice to compete in a lower weight division than usual training weight, theoretically to compete against smaller and weaker opponents. Like wrestlers and boxers, most lifters lose weight just prior to competition through dehydration and fasting. However, unlike wrestlers, studies of lifters report that many are at higher body-fat levels than necessary for an athlete, and could shed weight through loss of body fat. This could provide a long-term and safer way of making weight than previously practised, as well as ensure that lifters are in their most competitive weight division.

Read Chapters 3.1–3.4 to learn about setting and achieving an ideal body-fat and body-weight level.

### Making weight

Read Chapter 3.5 about making weight before competition. It warns of the disadvantages and dangers of dehydration and severe food restriction practices. Unlike wrestlers, most lifters may only need to use such drastic measures at three or four major competitions per year. Many compete in higher divisions or not at all outside these occasions. And unlike wrestlers and boxers, lifting events, being brief and power-related, are less likely to be impaired by dehydration and carbohydrate depletion than sparring events.

Nevertheless, there is a healthier and safer way to attack making weight. As explained in Chapter 3.5, you should keep within reach of your competition weight while in training by using sensible weight control techniques. The final kilo(s) can be shed easily in the later stages of preparation. No more saunas, spitting and diuretics!

### Lifestyle

Some strength athletes take advantage of their bulk when looking for employment, by taking jobs as 'bouncers' or security guards. On one level this can look like a handy part-time or full-time job, particularly if it is a night-time job that leaves you with your days free for training.

However, there are some traps involved with nocturnal work, particularly in places such as night clubs and discos. It can be difficult to maintain your nutrition goals and a proper sleep pattern. It is also tempting to get caught up in heavy alcohol intake, irregular meals based on convenience foods, and inadequate rest. Beware of throwing away your sporting goals because of this lifestyle.

It will take dedication and good planning to organise training and eating needs around a shift-work schedule. Be focused on your goals— read Chapters 1 and 2 to remind you of the principles of the optimum training diet.

### Blood lipids

Several studies of blood lipid measurements of throwers and lifters have reported high levels of cholesterol and triglycerides, and low levels of HDL-cholesterol (the protective form of cholesterol). This indicates an increased risk of coronary heart disease, and is in contrast to studies of endurance athletes that generally show quite low-risk profiles.

There are a number of reasons to explain the poor lipid profiles in these strength athletes. Firstly, some athletes are overweight, with body-fat levels that are obese even by community standards. Many athletes follow high-fat bulking up diets in search of high protein intakes. And finally, the use of anabolic steroids is known to disrupt lipid levels.

If you share any of these characteristics, particularly if you have a family history of heart disease, then a blood lipid screening should be undertaken. Even if the results are okay, you may be persuaded to change to a healthier lifestyle. There are other benefits to performance from following the principles of the optimum training diet in Chapters 1, 2 and 3. Be at your ideal body weight and body-fat level, and eat a high-energy diet that is high in carbohydrate and moderate in fat intake. High protein levels can easily be achieved with such a plan.


PROFILE: PAUL
*Get massive? Get organised!*

Paul weighed six kilograms less than the shotputter he wanted to be. At the end of last season he set a goal to be 95kg by his next competition, and his efforts over the following four months produced a gain of 1kg. For someone with his dedication this seemed slow progress. He trained hard in the gym, ate constantly and until he was uncomfortably full, and supplemented his diet with amino acids, herbal steroids and weight gain powder. Finally, in desperation, he consulted a dietitian.

The dietitian began by reviewing his goals. Had he set himself a realistic target? Had he allowed himself sufficient time to achieve this? Although a shotputter pays less penalty for having a high body-fat level that other athletes, Paul's target was to gain muscle (and strength) rather than pure body weight itself. His coach assured him that he had the body characteristics and a training program to bulk up well. It was theoretically possible to gain 1–2kg of lean body mass per month under circumstances such as this. Could the weak link be his diet?

Paul described a typical day of eating to the dietitian. A late but hearty breakfast of cereal, toast and eggs, followed by a session in the gym. Then it was home for a cooked lunch and off to afternoon lectures at the technical school. A quick dash to training, the evening workout, and home again to an evening of eating. His mother would have dinner number one ready when he walked in the door, and before he went to bed he would sit down to another sitting of leftovers and a weight-gain milkshake. His family marvelled that his evening meals totalled more than that of his mother, father and young sister combined.

On weekends, Paul explained that the routine changed due to his job as a 'bouncer' at a night club. Working 9pm–4am on Friday and Saturday nights meant having naps on Friday afternoon and between training sessions on Saturday. Sunday, a non-training day was spent catching up on lost sleep.

The dietitian suggested that Paul should keep a food diary during a typical week. The results came as a surprise to him, but it was quite easy to see his problem when it was written in black and white. Although he spent some parts of his day eating a lot, there were many hours that were quite devoid of food intake. Paul had many activities in his day—school, training, work and sleep. All these turned his attention away from food.

Weekends were a complete upheaval to his lifestyle, breaking up any routine that he might have developed during the week. Not only did he waste good 'eating time' during the day catching up on rest, but during the night at work he took only a couple of sandwiches to eat on his short rest-break, representing almost eight hours of wasted opportunity for energy intake.

The dietitian concluded that Paul's problem was simply an inadequate energy supply to support the maximum gain of muscle mass. She explained that an increased energy intake would bring with it increases in protein and all the other nutrients that were part of building new muscle. The solution was to find more efficient (and nutritious) ways to get kilojoules into his mouth, and the keys were planning and frequency.

Planning meant having foods on hand—for example, taking a supply of foods to eat on the way from school to the gym, and to eat while at work. Instead of taking a couple of rounds of sandwiches to the night club, Paul was advised to take a couple of frenchsticks made up into giant salad rolls. He could work his way through these, inch by inch, over the night.

High-energy drinks would also be part of the plan. The dietitian explained that there was nothing magical about the weight gain powder that he had bought from the health food shop. The trick was to use it more frequently, even three times a day between meals. She showed him several cheaper options in the form of homemade thickshakes and smoothies, using a less expensive commercial product or skim milk powder to boost the nutritional value. These drinks would be a mainstay on week-ends when Paul was trying to catch up with sleep. A snack and a drink could add up to plenty of kilojoules, and yet be quick and non-bulky so as to conserve his nap time. There is nothing worse than trying to sleep with a huge meal sitting uncomfortably in your stomach.

A meal plan was negotiated for Paul that consistently achieved six meals a day: breakfast as soon as he woke up, to be followed by a mid-morning milkshake before he left for training. Home for lunch, as before, but a couple of rolls and a thermos of his milk drink would accompany him to school for a snack between classes. In the evening he was to have two meals, one being the family dinner and the other a lighter snack and a high-energy fruit smoothie. This way he went to bed feeling less bloated, and ready for breakfast as soon as he woke up. A different, but nevertheless planned, routine was organised for weekends.

With his energy intake spread more evenly throughout the day, Paul was able to increase his total intake by almost 30 per cent. This kick-started his muscle gain program within a fortnight, and Paul achieved his target weight within six months. Since the herbal steroid and amino acid supplements did not seem to be part of the achievement, he was quite happy to abandon them along the way.

Paul found that his new body weight could only be maintained with dedication to his meal routine. For example, in celebrating the end of exams at school, he led a rather nomadic life for a fortnight—going out with friends at night and sleeping in later in the mornings. The scales showed a 2kg loss and reinforced the lesson that gains are made through a carefully planned diet rather than haphazard eating. Paul now appreciates that while he wants to continue his shotput career, he needs to treat his food intake with the same rigour and organisation that he shows in his training sessions.

PROFILE
*Food or pills?*

In 1984 an extensive dietary study was carried out on a group of national and international-level Australian Olympic weightlifters. The nineteen lifters were interviewed about their typical eating patterns and kept careful food diaries of a week's food and fluid intake. One of the most interesting features was the use of dietary supplements, with all lifters reporting daily use of supplements—often five or six different products at a time.

In order of popularity, supplements included multivitamin and B-vitamin formulas (used by 16 lifters), vitamin C (13 lifters), protein powders, liquids or tablets (12 lifters), calcium (12 lifters), 'vitamin' B15 (7 lifters), and herbal preparations including comfrey, ginseng and chlorophyll (7 lifters). Vitamin E supplements were taken by 6 lifters, electrolyte drinks or potassium tablets by 4 lifters, vitamin B12 (3 lifters), minerals such as iron or magnesium (2 lifters), amino acids (2 lifters), ATP powder (1 lifter) and ATP injections (1 lifter).

The reasons given for the use of these supplements were:

- that training increases nutritional requirements beyond the scope of dietary sources
- that certain supplements can directly improve training or competition performance.

The lifters quoted other lifters and health food shops as their major source of nutrition information, and those who had travelled to international competition were eager to swap secrets and supplements with Eastern Bloc athletes. This even extended to taking supplements with labels written in Russian and Bulgarian. Not knowing exactly what the contents were was no deterrent!

What can be said about these supplement practices? The first charge to be explored is that food cannot supply adequate nutrient levels for a weightlifter. The table below summarises the group average daily intake of selected vitamins and minerals, comparing intake from food with the intake supplied by supplements. To put this in perspective the recommended dietary intakes (RDIs) are presented.

**Nutrient intake from food and supplements compared in a group of 19 weightlifters**

| Nutrient | Number using supplements | Mean daily intake Supplements | Mean daily intake Food | RDI |
|---|---|---|---|---|
| Vitamin A | 10 | 2060µg | 2002µg | 750µg |
| Vitamin B1 (thiamin) | 15 | 93mg | 2.1mg | 1.5mg |
| Vitamin B2 (riboflavin) | 15 | 53mg | 3.5mg | 2.3mg |
| Vitamin B3 (niacin equiv.) | 15 | 122mg | 52.5mg | 24mg |
| Vitamin C | 16 | 1945mg | 199mg | 40mg |
| Iron | 10 | 8.0mg | 22.9mg | 7mg |
| Calcium | 15 | 473mg | 1567mg | 800mg |

Average daily intakes of protein and energy
Total intake of energy:  15 200 kJ/day (3640 Cal)
Contribution from supplements:  200 kJ/day (48 Cal)

Total intake of protein:  156g/day (= 1.8g/kg body weight)
Contribution from supplements:  6g/day

The lack of confidence in food seems unfounded according to these results. Although most weightifters chose a high-fat diet, the vitamin and mineral intakes from food sources exceeded the RDIs. Imagine what the results would look like if more nutritious lower-fat, higher carbohydrate diets were in place! The use of vitamin and mineral supplements provides a very haphazard nutrient intake profile. In some cases (e.g. thiamin and vitamin C) supplement intake provided nutrient levels far in excess of the RDIs. On the other hand, the intake of calcium and iron from supplements was small compared to that from food sources. And supplements were an insignificant source of energy and protein intake in this group. Hopefully a better appreciation of nutrient levels in food would help the weightlifters to re-think the need for protein, vitamin and mineral supplements. If nothing else, money could be saved on the supplements that provide an irrelevant nutrient supply.

Many of the other supplements used by these lifters fall into the nutritional ergogenic aid category (see Chapter 6), and into limbo with regard to proof that they work. It is not possible to answer the assertion that such supplements can assist training and competition performance, despite the 'scientific' theories put forward for some supplements. For example, it sounds clever to take ATP—getting right to the business end of the muscle's energy production. However, it is by no means certain that ATP, eaten or injected will make its way inside the muscle cell to where it is needed—in fact it seems highly unlikely. Therefore such supplements are unlikely to have a physiological effect.

Perhaps the major point of interest in the ergogenic aid supplements is to see how fashion changes. In 1984, the big sellers were B15 and herbal preparations. In the 1990s these have been replaced by amino acids and Frac. Even without the verdict of scientific trials, what does the swing in (sports) public opinion tell us?

While these lifters may have enjoyed a psychological boost from their use of supplements, it is not possible to tell whether this translated into better performances. It would be interesting to see whether the weightlifters would change these practices, if their information sources were sports scientists and nutritionists, rather than health food shops and each other.

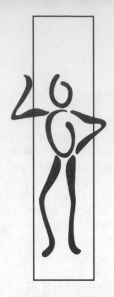

# Body building

Bodybuilders are primarily concerned not with strength or other parameters of athletic prowess, but with their physique. Muscular definition, balanced development of different body parts and symmetry of development are the criteria upon which bodybuilding competitions are judged. Not all bodybuilders compete, however. Many simply enjoy the challenge of improving their physique and appearance through training and diet.

### Training

The year of a competitive bodybuilder is broken into three phases. In the off-season, training is targeted at bulking up, or increasing overall muscle size. The result is that most bodybuilders are well over competition weight, and body-fat levels can be relatively high. As the competition season approaches, bodybuilders begin to 'cut up'—aiming to lose body fat in order to increase muscle definition without losing muscle mass or size. Finally, in the days or week prior to competition, bodybuilders undertake special methods to achieve cosmetic changes that will make their bodies appear 'pumped', with clearly defined muscularity and vascularity. Bodybuilders who do not take part in competitions may simply train to bulk up.

The exact training methods used by bodybuilders are diverse and dramatic, and there are as many enthusiastically recommended programs as there are articles in bodybuilding magazines. In general, both elite and recreational bodybuilders can spend many hours in the gym each day, usually following 'split routines' where different parts of the body are trained at different sessions. Training typically involves three to five exercises for each of the six major muscle groups (chest, back, arms, legs, shoulders and abdomen). Each exercise normally comprises three to six sets of lifts or repetitions. Bodybuilders usually perform a greater number of repetitions per set (6–15) than do power and weight lifters (1–5) since this provides for greater muscular hypertrophy.

In the cutting-up phase many bodybuilders incorporate more aerobic exercise into their programs to help reduce body-fat levels.

## Competition

There are three stages of judging involved in bodybuilding competitions: the structural round in which all competitors are judged on stage together while in relaxed pose, the individual posing routine in which competitors display their own routine of poses lasting about two minutes, and the compulsory poses which are judged comparatively.

Depending on the number of age or weight divisions, judging can take six hours or more.

## Physical characteristics

The physical characteristics of bodybuilders are striking and well-known—almost needing no explanation. Bodybuilders have a large total body weight due to pronounced muscle development. Depending on the time of the year, body fat levels can vary from normal-high during the bulking-up phase, to minimum skinfold sums during the competition phase.

## Other comments

The world of bodybuilding is flamboyant. Bodybuilders have a unique lifestyle and beliefs that are often viewed as bizarre and even unattractive by those outside the sport. They are a close-knit group, with information being spread pervasively and persuasively through their circles, by word of mouth and through bodybuilding magazines. Perhaps the most-well known of these is Joe Weider's *Muscle and Fitness* magazine, which has a readership of over six million people, worldwide. Understandably, those at the top of the empire have great power to shape the beliefs, as well as the muscles, of those below.

Most of the 'science' of bodybuilding comes from other bodybuilders—champions maybe, but non-scientists nevertheless. While there are a few bodybuilders or followers of the sport with legitimate scientific qualifications, there are others who quote qualifications that are at best unorthodox and unrecognised. Thus, many bizarre and occasionally dangerous practices have been used and promoted in bodybuilding, including the use of drugs.

Probably more than any other sport, bodybuilding has placed emphasis on the role of nutrition in performance and bodybuilders are unique in their fastidious attention to food. However, not all the nutrition philosophies—and there are as many as there are training philosophies—agree with established scientific views.

It is hard to compete against the typical bodybuilder's nutritional beliefs and practices. For a start, it is hard to compete against the powerful communication and merchandising networks, and the testimonials of the champions. And, sadly, it is sometimes hard to measure up against the undeniable results that can be gained through the use of anabolic steriods, or other unsafe practices. Healthy or safe dietary practices which are offered as an alternative are at a clear disadvantage if they cannot match these results. Nevertheless, it is hoped that with time and with access to scientific and health-minded nutrition information, at least some bodybuilders will make the transition.

### Common nutrition issues

#### Who is a nutrition expert?

Almost every bodybuilding magazine carries a number of articles in which top competitors share their dietary and training secrets. Other articles are written by people with 'scientific' qualifications which do not fit within the mainstream academic program. Who should you listen to? How do you know who the real experts are?

Most people, athletes or otherwise, give each other advice or comments about their diets, and it has been suggested that some nutrition 'experts' have as their only qualification the fact that they have eaten food almost every day of their lives. The ideal nutrition advice is something that has been rigorously studied and tested, and the results scrutinised by a variety of objective scientists. And it will probably be found to complement the general nutrition guidelines for health and athletic performance, rather than oppose them.

In Chapter 5 the basis of scientific proof was discussed in relation to dietary supplements. This theme can be extended to all nutrition issues. Testimonials from successful athletes and scientific theories can provide the material for ideas to be tested. However, until the idea is adequately tested, no judgement can or should be made. Many of the dietary philosophies of bodybuilders remain on the drawing board, awaiting attention. Interestingly, they can't all work, since some ideas flatly contradict others.

What are the problems with using practices that are not yet tested and approved? In some cases, there may be no major disadvantages and even some benefits—the practice may actually work, you may get a psychological edge from your belief in it, or you may simply enjoy the feeling of being part of the scene. On the other hand, some dietary practices are expensive, and some are unhealthy—even dangerous.

When trying to evaluate dietary advice or the credentials of the nutrition expert promoting it, the checklist following may be useful. Read all the articles in your bodybuilding magazine with interest, but learn to distinguish the columns that carry more weighty material. You'll probably notice that some magazines are now regularly including information from more legitimate sources.

---

## CHECKLIST TO EVALUATE DIETARY ADVICE

- What recognised qualifications does the nutrition 'expert' have?
  Check with a sports dietitian if you are unsure.

- Does it promise results that are too good to be true?
  They probably are!

- Is the advice based only on an idea or case histories—regardless of which famous athlete swears by the advice or how 'scientific' the theory sounds?

- Have the ideas been scientifically tested and reported in a reputable journal?
  These journals accept only those studies that have been adequately conducted and the results handled by proper statistical methods. Check with a sports dietitian if you're not sure.

- Is the advice generally compatible with healthy nutrition guidelines, or is the advice supported by recognised nutrition authorities?
  Again, check with a sports dietitian.

- Is anyone going to make money from this advice?

---

*Nutritional ergogenic aids*

Studies of bodybuilders have reported that, despite nutrient intake from food being up to 400 per cent of the recommended dietary intake levels, there is widespread use of dietary supplements. Numerous supplements are taken in large doses, sometimes with nutrient intakes reaching levels that are regarded as toxic. Other supplements do not provide nutrients, but large doses of strange and rare substances found in food.

173

Apart from the advice or observation of everyone else in the gym, the best support for supplements comes from bodybuilding magazines. Magazines can carry up to 30 pages of advertisements in each edition, not to mention unpaid testimonials and articles which all proclaim the virtues of various products—from traditional favourites such as weight gain powders and vitamins to the latest trends in amino acids and Frac. The supplements promise a variety of wonderful achievements—some claiming to help you 'get massive', others to promote fat mobilisation and loss to help you 'get ripped', and still others to give you more energy in training. Some supplements are directly promoted as an alternative to steroids, dramatically claiming that they will pass all drug tests.

It should come as no surprise that the supplement industry makes millions of dollars from bodybuilders—and makes millions of dollars *for* some bodybuilders. Interestingly, a huge supplement range is marketed by the same person who owns and publishes the largest-selling body-building magazines. Cynics might see the magazine almost as a manufacturer's catalogue, although the advertisements are more powerful and emotive than the junkmail that you normally get in your letterbox.

Chapter 6 gives the low-down on supplements, with most body-building supplements falling into the nutritional ergogenic aid group. The bottom line is that we don't know whether such supplements work, since they have not been adequately tested. By the same token, we can't be sure that they do not work. Whether you experiment for yourself is an individual decision, but realise that you may be paying to be a guinea pig in an uncontrolled experiment.

Meanwhile, there are *some* dietary supplements that can be of proven help to bodybuilders. Bulking up often requires a bodybuilder to consume more food energy than is practical or comfortable. High-energy, nutritious fluids can be a useful way to boost energy intake—see Chapter 3.6. Although you can make your own low-fat milk shakes and smoothies, supplements such as weight-gain powders can help to fortify a drink with extra kilojoules and nutrients. Note that you do not need a high-protein formula, but rather a high-carbohydrate complete nutrition formula.

If you check the price of bodybuilding supplements, you will find that the cheapest commercial supplements are pharmaceutical products such as Sustagen or Exceed Sports Nutrition Supplement. They are also formulated with a balanced nutrient profile that mimics recommended dietary intakes, rather than 'special' ingredients such as gamma-oryzanol, free-form amino acids and carnitine.

### Bulking-up

While there are many variations on a theme, the typical bodybuilder undertakes a rigid and quite unusual dietary pattern during the bulking-up phase of training. Typically, bodybuilders believe in high-energy, high-protein diets. The traditional high-protein diet is also high in fat, since these nutrients are often found simultaneously in foods. However, in recent years the role of carbohydrate as a muscle fuel has been recognised. Thus the contemporary bodybuilding diet is now high in protein, moderate-to-high in carbohydrate and low in fat. Some competitors make these ratios more extreme.

It is not just the principles of the diet that can be rigid. Many bodybuilders set themselves a narrow range of foods, and an unchanging meal plan to meet their dietary targets. Many make meals from large quantities of a few chosen foods—particularly low-fat, high-protein types, and repeat the same meal plan day after day. In fact, you can often pick a bodybuilder not just from their muscle-bound appearance, but from the contents of their shopping trolleys. Look for lots of chicken breasts, cans of tuna (water-packed), cartons of eggs (they eat only the whites) and skim milk powder. For carbohydrates, rice cakes, rice and pasta are popular.

The high-energy diet is eaten in a series of meals, often six to eight over the day. This is a practical way to ensure that large energy intakes are managed, and may also maximise the metabolic gains from food. See Chapter 2.7 for more details.

Chapter 3.6 summarises the principles of gaining muscle mass: the right parents, the right training, and a diet that supplies adequate energy and all other nutrients. Protein requirements for maximum muscle gain have long been debated, with the current consensus being that they are likely to be elevated above normal (sedentary) requirements, but still within the range of a high-energy diet of normal protein-to-energy ratio.

Nutrition experts argue that even the highest protein intake that can be justified scientifically, that is 1.5–2.0g/kg of body weight per day, can be achieved in a high-energy diet. However, studies of bodybuilders report that actual intakes are often twice as high, with protein being elevated to more than 20 per cent of total energy intake. Because many bodybuilders are unable to translate food into nutrients, they may be unaware of their total protein loads. Some will even add a high-protein supplement to a diet that already exceeds the level of possible protein utilisation.

While bodybuilders are to be congratulated on their dietary concern and motivation, there are perhaps three areas for improvement of present typical meal plans:

• Protein intakes need not be as high as often achieved.

• By virtue of high-energy intakes and the nutritious choice of foods, the vitamin and mineral intakes of most bodybuilders are also expected to exceed the recommended dietary intake levels. With this confidence, some bodybuilders may re-think their use of vitamin supplements.

- There are many ways of choosing and enjoying foods to achieve a healthy dietary intake. Most bodybuilders could enjoy a greater range and flexibility with foods, including greater variety and versatility at meals.

### Cutting-up

The length and severity of the cutting-up phase will vary between bodybuilders. Some competitors remain in shape during the bulking-up phase and leave adequate time before competition for a consistent and moderate rate of body-fat loss (0.5–1.0kg/week). Other body-builders set out to lose large amounts of body fat in a short time (2kg/week)—perhaps because they have budgeted only a short contest preparation period, or because they believe that dramatic weight loss will achieve a more dramatic 'ripped' or 'shredded' appearance. Unfortunately, rapid weight loss has the disadvantage of sacrificing muscle mass.

Typically, body-fat loss is achieved by increased aerobic exercise and restriction of dietary energy. Some bodybuilders cut back on the total quantity of all foods, while other severely restrict carbohydrate intake. In any case, the typical cutting-up diet is even more regimented and inflexible than the bulking-up phase. Certain supplements are promoted as 'fat burners'—particularly carnitine—and may be added to the weight loss diet.

For a guide to safe and healthy body-fat loss, which aims to preserve total nutritional goals and minimise loss of muscle mass, read Chapter 3.3. It is both unnecessary and a disadvantage to become too rigid and restrictive in dietary energy intake and variety.

### The pre-competition diet

A bodybuilder aims to enter the contest with his or her muscles looking 'pumped' and fully defined, with clear detail of the striations and vascularity in each muscle. A number of techniques are used to achieve the last fine-tuning. Many bodybuilders carbo-load over the last week, depleting their muscles of carbohydrate over the first part of the week, and switching to a high-carbohydrate diet over the last couple of days. The aim is to store extra glycogen (and water) in the muscles, making them look 'pumped' and massive. There are many stories of when and how to achieve loading, without overshooting the mark, and making the muscles look too smooth.

Fluid and electrolyte balance is also manipulated in the last couple of days, with the aim of dehydrating the skin and making it appear tightly stretched over the muscles. Techniques include fluid and sodium restriction, and the use of diuretics and potassium supplements. Many of these practices are harmful and there have been stories of bodybuilders collapsing on stage due to dehydration and electrolyte imbalances—for example, Albert Beckles in 1988.

The best advice is to experiment with your pre-contest strategies to find a loading practice that puts you at your best—not just in appearance but in overall health. Avoid techniques that are severe and drug-based.

### Blood cholesterol levels

Studies of bodybuilders have reported blood cholesterol and triglyceride levels that are unfavourable in terms of heart disease risk. Low levels of HDL-cholesterol—the 'good' cholesterol that helps to protect against coronary heart disease—are a particular concern.

In the case of old-fashioned bodybuilders, an unfavourable blood-lipid profile may be partly explained by a high-fat intake. However, the major cause of such disturbed cholesterol levels is steroid abuse, perhaps sentencing long-term users to a greater risk of heart disease. Fortunately, the abnormal cholesterol levels appear to be quickly reversed when steroids are discontinued.

## PROFILES
### Exploring the myths

Although well-meaning advice is given by one bodybuilder to another, there are many myths and misconceptions spread through body-building circles.

Dear Muscle-Magazine,

I am the original 10 stone weakling—65 kg to be exact. I'm tired of every-one laughing at my puny body and kicking sand in my face at the beach, so I've decided to do something about it once and for all. I joined Silver's Gym last month and got a weight training program written for me. Can you advise me what sort of diet I need to help me to bulk up.

Ronald

*Dear Ronald,*

*Congratulations on joining the sport of bodybuilding. I used to be just like you, so take heart. Of course it has taken me many years to build up to this level, but you are right about the importance of diet. Superior nutrition was my secret weapon in winning the Mr World title last year—it's the only way to push yourself over the edge.*

*I have refined this plan over a number of years and stick closely to it when I am bulking up. A typical day's menu is:*

*Breakfast: 10 egg whites + 1 egg yolk, made into an omelette*
*100g oats + 50g raisins + cup skim milk*
*Meal 2: (after training) 200g tin of tuna (water packed)*
*200g boiled rice*
*cup of broccoli*

Lunch: *250g lean steak*
*1 cup cooked pasta*
Meal 4: *250g lean steak*
*100g boiled rice*
Dinner: *200g tin of tuna (water packed)*
*100g boiled rice*
Meal 6: *10 egg whites cooked into omelette*
*2 rice cakes*

*I change this round by having different green vegies or salad each day, and by interchanging chicken breasts and the lean steak. This diet is extremely low in fat and high in protein and carbs. Good luck with your training,*
*Mr World*

*Comment* Photos of Mr World attest that he is indeed massive, with the identifiable factors in his success being years of hard training and the right genetic potential. Mr World's diet will not achieve a similar success for Ron in the absence of these ingredients. It is difficult to predict how much diet has contributed to Mr World's physique. Certainly, a diet that is inadequate in energy, carbohydrate, protein or any of the vitamins and minerals involved in growth and exercise metabolism, will hold back the progress and results of training. But can extra protein and vitamins increase muscle mass? Current scientific knowledge says no.

An analysis of Mr World's typical daily intake reveals the following estimations: 14 060kJ (3355 Cals), 350g of protein, 330g of carbohydrate, and 77g of fat. Protein intake provides over 40 per cent of his total energy intake—slightly more than his carbohydrate intake. Mr World weighs in at 100kg, giving him a protein intake of about 3.5g/kg body weight. If Ron were to eat the same diet, he would achieve a protein intake exceeding 5g/kg/day. Conventional science says that it is not possible to utilise such high protein intakes. At best, this protein becomes an expensive energy source. At worst, there may be health penalties to pay for chronic intakes of such high protein loads.

Read Chapters 1 and 2 to find the principles and food aspects of healthy training nutrition. Mr World's diet is not really as high in carbohydrates as he imagines—less than 3.5g/kg/day to fuel his workouts. He might be surprised to find that swapping some of his protein budget for carbohydrate energy will increase his training performance. Above all, it is unnecessary to maintain such a rigidness with meal choices, and to eat the same thing day in, day out. Variety adds nutritional depth as well as food enjoyment.

Dear Muscle-Magazine,
Can you give me some tips on good nutrition for the intermediate bodybuilder? I want to be a champion like Arnold someday,
Larry

*Dear Larry,*
*   The best advice I can give you about diet is to keep it simple and natural.*
*This way you won't overload your body's digestive system, and will get full*
*value from the food you eat. Have many small meals rather than large meals.*
*Eat food raw and whole as much as possible—for example, raw vegetables*
*and salad rather than cooked vegetables, whole meat rather than minced*
*meat, whole fruit rather than juices.*
*   Don't eat too many foods at the one time. It is better to have two or three*
*different foods at a meal and another three at your next meal than to bombard*
*your intestines with too many foods all at once. The worst combinations are*
*protein foods mixed with acidic foods such as oranges, and protein mixed*
*with carbohydrate foods. Digestive enzyme supplements are an excellent aid*
*if you have already overstrained your system. Regards,*
*   Mr Galaxy*

*Comment*   The human body has remarkable powers of adaptation,
otherwise there would be no rewards from training. Your digestive
system is quite sophisticated and well-equipped to handle the challenges of a varied diet. Think back to your school biology lessons—
you may remember that your small intestines work like a long conveyor
belt. Food is passed down its length, firstly being broken down to its
smallest molecules, and then passing to the special site programmed
to absorb particular nutrients. Everything is well organised—various
sections are specialised for each duty, so there is no worry about
overloading or overstressing the system. Additional 'digestive enzymes'
are not needed, and anyway the popular supplements marketed for
this purpose are unlikely to pass though the acidic stomach environment without being inactivated.

In Chapter 1 the benefits of food variety were discussed, including
the advantages of mixing and matching foods at the same meal. In
general, nutrients and food factors interact to improve the nutritional
quality of the meal. Rather than follow Mr Galaxy's advice, Larry should
aim to include many different foods in each meal. This makes for
more interesting and enjoyable eating as well. Despite the publicity,
there is *no* danger in combining protein and carbohydrate—it already
happens inside foods such as bread, pasta and rice. Concern over
acidic foods is also unfounded since the acid content of the stomach
far outstrips any dietary source.

In general, foods that are minimally processed or cooked will maintain their maximum nutrient value. Thus it is good to include foods
that can be eaten raw or in as natural a state as possible. However,
it is not necessary or even helpful to insist that all foods are left raw
and whole. There are many ways to prepare and cook foods that
minimise the loss of nutritional value or the addition of less desirable
compounds such as fat, sugar or salt. Practise moderation and flexibility
in all aspects of nutrition.

Dear Muscle-Magazine,
   Help! I'm confused. First I read that bodybuilders should eat high protein diets, then I read that they should eat plenty of carbs. What's the correct advice?
   Laura

*Dear Laura,*
   *Yes, there is a lot of conflicting information about this area of nutrition. My own experiments have allowed me to work out a solution—at least one that works for me. I favour the high protein look since that helps me to look hard and chiselled. However, when I say high protein I don't mean fish and chicken. I mean beef—two to three pounds a day.*
   *Beef is meat muscle. It's already full of glycogen, so you don't have to eat much other carbohydrate. Besides, the glycogen is already processed, so it doesn't need to go through digestion and absorption. It can go straight to your muscles.*
   *I have used this approach in my training this year and the results of the Ms Globe contest speak for themselves.*
   *Ms Globe*

*Comment*   As interesting as Ms Globe's theories sound, they contradict both food composition information and the laws of human physiology. There is negligible carbohydrate in meat, whether beef, chicken or fish. Meat is technically animal muscle, accounting for its high protein content. However, muscle glycogen stores do not account for a great mass of carbohydrate—at least not in the quantity of meat that you are likely to eat at the one time. Additionally, most of the glycogen is broken down in the slaughtering process.

Even if glycogen could be consumed in appreciable amounts, it would have to go through the same digestion processes as any carbohydrate in food. You body will not discriminate and send it to re-form in the muscle either. It will simply add to the body carbohydrate pool, and its fate will be decided according to the body's immediate requirements.

If you are still confused about the body's requirements for protein and carbohydrate, go back to Chapter 2 (sections 2.2 and 2.3). A high-energy diet will be high in all nutrients, but for athletes in heavy training the most important fuel source is dietary carbohydrate.

Dear Muscle-Magazine,
   I have been training for three years and plan to enter competition soon. I have very little spare money and want to know if it is possible to get to the top without taking supplements. Also, what supplements are the best value?
   David

*Dear David*
   *I sympathise with you. The more advanced you become, the more important and significant is the role of nutrition. The blasting training sessions typical of champion bodybuilders place a great stress on normal nutrition*

*stores. Without adequate nutrients you will not get maximal gains. Supplements are your best health insurance, since they will provide all the nutrients needed in quantities not possible though ordinary foods. My own program includes Crash Weight Gain powder, amino acids, megaformula multivitamins, gamma-oryzanol and inosine. When cutting up I use extra doses of carnitine.*

*If you are on a tight budget, go for the Crash Weight Gain formula and a multivitamin product. When taken as directed and in conjunction with your workouts, it can help you to gain up to a pound a day. I use it in my training to bulk up quickly. You can do the same.*

*Mr International*

**Comment**  Read about supplements in Chapter 6! It is not possible to gain a pound of muscle—or even fat—each day. Set your sights on a more realistic goal. The Crash Weight Gain formula, being a high-energy nutritious drink, can help you to boost energy intake while on a bulking up program (see Chapter 3.6), but there are less expensive ways to achieve the same result. The least expensive commercial supplements of this type are the pharmaceutical brands. However, you can make a cheaper version yourself by blending together skim milk plus extra skim milk powder, banana or other fruit, and some ice cubes.

Optional extras are low-fat yoghurt or perhaps low-fat icecream.

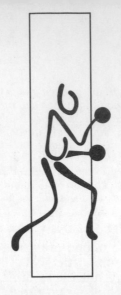

# Wrestling and boxing

Wrestling and boxing are male-only combative sports which share a similar competition structure in terms of having both weight divisions, and a marked division between amateur and professional codes.

There are ten divisions in wrestling, from light flyweight (below 48kg) to heavyweight plus (100–130kg). Boxing is run by a number of governing bodies, with at least eleven or twelve weight divisions depending on the federation. In general, divisions range from light flyweight (below 48kg) to heavyweight (above 80kg).

The duration of an amateur wrestling bout has undergone many changes, and is currently contested over one five-minute round. An amateur boxing match is fought over three 3-minute rounds. Professional bouts in both sports can be up to fifteen 3-minute rounds. Both sports feature relatively short bursts of high-intensity anaerobic effort against a background of continuous low-intensity activity. Although aerobic fitness is important to both wrestlers and boxers in helping recovery between bursts, it is the ability to generate muscular force quickly that is the primary requirement for successful competition.

### Training

The training of wrestlers and boxers will depend on their mode of competition, whether in weekly bouts, in multi-day tournaments, or as a single fight. In the latter situation, for example in the case of a professional boxer, there may be long periods between fights during which time specific training and even general fitness work may be suspended or reduced.

However in the lead-up to a competition, wrestlers and boxers train daily, supplementing skill and technique sessions with various forms of aerobic training such as running and skipping. Weight training may be undertaken to increase muscular strength and power, but becomes less important just before or during the competition phase.

In the competition phase, attention turns to making weight, and the athlete may increase the aerobic training load to help reduce body-fat levels. Often, food and fluid restriction and other rapid weight-loss techniques are employed to assist in achieving weigh-in targets.

Where weekly competition is undertaken, then a mini-cycle will operate, with heavier training during the first part of the week, and weight-loss activities dominating the end of the week prior to the weekend match.

## Competition

Competition may be organised as a single bout, a weekly competition, or a multi-day tournament. Weigh-in is normally completed on the morning of a competition, which in the case of a major fight, may leave eight hours to rehydrate and prepare for the evening bout.

Recovery from bouts—and from repeated efforts to 'make weight'—is especially important in multi-day tournaments and weekly competitions, and athletes who fight at their natural weight have an advantage over athletes who must continually cut weight. In single fights, the effects of cutting weight may increase with the length of the bout, and a fighter may try to force an early conclusion before his stamina is tested.

## Physical characteristics

There are a wide range of body sizes seen in these combative sports, with the weight divisions attempting to level out the physical inequalities between competitors. Top wrestlers and boxers tend to low body-fat levels, trying to maximise power and strength for their weight limit. In the heavyweight divisions of boxing, higher body-fat levels are seen.

## Common nutrition issues

### Training nutrition

Many wrestlers and boxers do not set themselves a routine training diet. Rather they move between extremes of eating everything and eating nothing depending on the phase of their competition. This may happen over a weekly cycle for those in a competition season, or on a more extended level for those who compete sporadically in major fights. Clearly this is not ideal for either nutritional status or weight control.

Why not take a completely different and more long-term view of your sport and your diet? Read Chapters 1 and 2 for an overview of the healthy training diet. A balanced and stable program will be better for body and soul, avoiding the physical and mental stress that goes with the current practice of jumping from one extreme to another.

### Choosing a fighting weight

Combative athletes choose their fighting weight for many reasons, few of which are based on healthiness and optimum performance level. In the case of professional athletes it may be to chase an opponent or a title, and these athletes often fight at a number of weight divisions depending on what is on offer. Wrestlers may select their weight division because it is the only available spot on the school or club wrestling team. Adolescents may be chosen or certified at one weight division at the beginning of a season, and then fail to take into account growth and weight gain in the subsequent months.

There are two philosophies, integral to combative sports, that continue to support these decisions. The first is the belief that it is necessary to gain an advantage of strength, speed and leverage by fighting against a smaller opponent. By coming down from a weight that is above the limits of their weight division, wrestlers and boxers feel that they have achieved this goal. Of course, the advantage is wiped if their opponent has done exactly the same thing, and if the methods used to cut weight actually impair performance.

The second factor is the acceptance of rapid weight-loss techniques. Not only have they become a means to an end, but they have become ingrained in the language and the culture of these sports. The restricted eating, the excessive training and the saunas are almost part of the romance of being a wrestler. They have become a shared experience or common interest that bonds people within the sport—despite the disadvantages to health and performance. Read the account below to see just how institutionalised these practices have become, and the price that must be paid in return.

Numerous calls have been made to clean up this aspect of wrestling and boxing, particularly where adolescents are involved and particularly where competition (and therefore weight-loss practices) are frequent. The first step is to set realistic competition weights, based on a weight and body-fat level that is healthy and achievable for the athlete. For growing adolescents this may need to be continually reassessed. If you have body fat to spare there may be leeway for weight loss. However, if you are already at a low body-fat level you should think carefully about the weight division you choose. See Chapter 3 for a more detailed discussion.

## Making weight

The study of the wrestlers below highlights the wrong way to approach weight-limits and weight loss. The physical and psychological disadvantages, both short-term and long-term, are clearly outlined. From a distance, it seems obvious that better selection of weight divisions and healthier weight-loss or weight-control programs would benefit combative sports, both in presenting athletes at their peak for competition, and in reducing the negative side-effects in general. Of course, it is hard when you are close to a sport to see the total perspective, or to see how major changes in attitude can come about. Nevertheless, it is up to all those involved—coaches, athletes and administrators—to slowly push for change.

Read Chapter 3 for a clearer account of healthy weight-loss, including both long-term weight control and last-minute fine-tuning before a competition. If you can maintain a general training weight within a kilogram of so of your competition target, it is possible to 'tickle' off the last grams without fuss or detriment (Chapter 3.5). This can be practised both in a weekly competition, and as in the case of Ross below, for a special one-off fight. While these healthier techniques might strip combative sports of some of their tradition and some of the locker-room talk—who really needs it? The wrestler's world can sound brave and wonderful in books and films, but the reality of diuretics, induced vomiting and sweat-boxes is hardly glamourous.

PROFILE
## The life of a college wrestler

Amateur wrestling has a large following in high schools and colleges in the USA. Typically, the wrestling season involves weekly competition, with athletes certifying in a weight class that is below their off-season weight in order to gain a theoretical advantage over smaller opponents. Weigh-ins are conducted before each competition bout, requiring a weekly struggle to cut weight to the competition target. Following a match, wrestlers typically consume large amounts of food and drink, relaxing their end-of-week restrictions and gaining excess kilos that must be shed by the next weigh-in. This pattern of weight loss and regain is repeated throughout the competition season.

The rapid loss of body weight is achieved though one or more of the following: very restricted nutrition, artificial means of dehydration, and excessive exercise. A survey of large number of high school and college wrestlers was recently conducted to paint a picture of the typical lifestlye involved.

The mean age of the wrestlers was sixteen years (high school) and twenty years (college). The average age at which cutting weight began was fourteen years. On average, the high school wrestlers reported cutting weight nine times a season, with the college wrestlers needing to do this fifteen times in their competitive year. Weekly weight fluctuations ranged from 3–9kg/week for the college athletes, with smaller amounts being reported by their high school counterparts. Looking over their careers, a third of the college wrestlers estimated that they had to cut 5kg at least 100 times, and 20 per cent reported that they had lost 5–10 kg between 20 and 50 times.

Details of the weight-loss methods used by wrestlers were provided. About a third of the group dehydrated using a sauna or rubber/plastic suit while exercising, at least once a week. Eighty percent restricted fluids at least once a week, with half this number restricting fluids three to four times each week. Food was restricted by half the group, three or four times a week, and daily by a fifth of the wrestlers. More than half the group completely fasted once a week. Vomiting, laxatives and diuretics were used by smaller numbers on a less frequent basis.

Most of the wrestlers reported that it was difficult to make weight, and reported severe fatigue (75 per cent), anger (66 per cent), anxiety (33 per cent), feelings of isolation (23 per cent), depression (24 per cent) and low self-esteem (12 per cent). They reported that they were often or always preoccupied with foods, and many felt out of control with eating.

Apart from the psychological problems and the unhappiness associated with cutting weight, there are physical effects on both health and performance that need to be considered. Rapid weight loss is achieved through loss of body water, glycogen and perhaps protein (muscle). There is insufficient time between weigh-in and the event in most sports for adequate recovery of fluid and fuel stores to take place, leaving the athlete at a competitive disadvantage. During the training week, chronic weight-loss efforts may also take their toll.

While dehydration may not impair strength for short-duration exercise of seconds, it has been shown to impair exercise of two to three minutes or more and to decrease recovery, thus reducing performance in most competition situations. In the training situation, lack of concentration and loss of muscular endurance will interfere with training for improved fitness and skill acquisition. Loss of strength may eventually result if muscle is sacrificed.

Some of the weight-loss techniques also cause other side-effects, such as the loss of electrolytes with vomiting and laxative use. Restrictive diets will eventually impair nutritional status, perhaps with vitamin and mineral deficiencies, and with an effect on energy metabolism. Weight cycling is believed to depress energy requirements, making it even more difficult to shed real body fat.

Just because these weight-loss techniques are an accepted part of wrestling, does not mean they are acceptable practices. It is hoped that with time and education, a fairer approach will be taken in such sports—fairer to the basic idea of matching equal opponents in competition, and fairer to the athlete in allowing him to reach optimum health and performance.

PROFILE: ROSS
*Fighting fit and light*

Ross consulted a sports dietitian when things looked bleak twelve weeks before his next title fight. Life had been a little up and down in the past year. Twice he had had title fights cancelled, although the last time—a last-minute cancellation—it was probably a blessing in disguise. With four weeks to go, he was still 6 kg overweight, and had been making poor progress with either his training or his weight.

It was hard, when the competition schedule was so infrequent and so uncertain, to keep himself motivated. After his last fight nine months ago, he had been so glad that the battle was over (both in the ring and with the bathroom scales each morning) that he had slipped gladly into a life of sloth and gluttony for a couple of months. This had left a legacy of an additional 9kg above his weight division, a figure that had gone up and down between the training come-backs and false starts. Losing weight was becoming increasingly harder with each fight, and Ross was becoming tired of the pressure it put on his career. Could a dietitian get him down to 59kg in twelve weeks, without costing him his sanity and his sweet tooth?

The dietitian firstly assessed Ross's body-fat levels to determine what excess baggage he had to shed. With skinfold levels of 92mm, she agreed that body fat could be safely lost. A loss of 50mm of body fat could well equate with the 9kg that he needed to lose, meaning that Ross need not jeopardise muscle mass to get down near his fighting weight. She listened to his training program, and advised him that a slow but steady rate of loss would be needed—not only to ensure that fat was lost preferentially, but to ensure that adequate carbohydrate and nutrient intake would be supplied to support his exercise needs. Eight kilograms in twelve weeks would be hard work, but could be achieved without the usual problems of fatigue, irritability, and mental stress. His wife and his coach were also pleased with this news.

The dietitian devised a menu plan of 7500 kJ (1800 Cals), including a high carbohydrate intake, plenty of nutrient-rich foods and a sprinkling of 'treat' foods that helped to put a sparkle in his day. The outline of this plan is presented in the table below. Ross's wife worked with the dietitian to prepare different recipes and variations on the theme. Ross was astounded—he'd never lost weight before without

187

**Typical day's eating for Ross (boxer)—weight loss diet**

| | |
|---|---|
| Breakfast (after training) | Medium bowl of wholegrain cereal<br>Skim milk<br>2 slices wholegrain toast + jam<br>Unsweetened fruit juice or piece of fruit<br>Tea with skim milk |
| Lunch | Sandwich or roll—wholemeal bread, no margarine<br>Small amount of chicken, cottage cheese, salmon<br>or lean roast meat<br>Plenty of salad<br>Fruit scone or muffin—unbuttered<br>Low-joule drink |
| Afternoon tea (prior to training) | Low-joule drink<br>Piece of fruit |
| Tea | Lean meat, fish or chicken—100–120g serve<br>Cup of wholemeal rice, pasta or large potato<br>Plenty of other vegetables or salad<br>Medium serve of fruit salad or low-fat fruit yoghurt |

Once a week treat of chocolate bar or icecream in cone

Energy: 7500–8000 kilojoules (1800–2000 Cals)
Carbohydrate: 320g (60–65% of energy)
Protein: 90g (20% of energy)
Fat: 25–30g (15–20% of energy)
Vitamins and minerals: all above RDI level

having to face endless nights of steamed fish and boiled chicken. He felt more energetic in training than ever before, and enjoyed his sweet treats without feeling guilty.

After four weeks he had lost 4kg (skinfolds down by 18mm), and at eight weeks was within 3kg of his weigh-in limit (skinfolds down by a total of 35mm). At the beginning of the title fight week, he was within 1.5kg of his target (weight 60.5kg, skinfolds 47mm), and under the dietitian's instructions he began to move into competition mode to shake off the last grams.

For the four days until the weigh-in, Ross restricted his salt intake, making sure that body fluid accumulation would be avoided. All salt was cut from his meals (pepper helped to flavour the cooking), and he was careful to avoid salty foods such as cheese, nuts, chips, processed meats and salted crackers (not that these foods had been part of his diet for a while). On the Thursday, he ate his normal breakfast, and then switched to drinking a Sustagen low-fat milkshake for lunch, afternoon tea and dinner. He woke up on the Friday morning feeling nervous, but light and trim—and his flat stomach showed-off the ripplemarks of all his recent training.

Weigh-in was conducted before Ross had eaten or drunk anything, and the scales rewarded him with a reading of 58.7kg. For the remainder of the day, he rested and ate light snacks of carbohydrate foods, topping up his fluid levels at frequent intervals. A final light meal was eaten at 4.30pm, about three hours before he had to step into the ring.

And the fight was great. He felt confident and strong both physically and mentally. Hearing that his opponent had spent two hours in the sauna that morning before weighing-in had given him a great psychological boost. He remembered all the times that he had resorted to that himself, and how dreadful he had felt on the occasion that he had taken a diuretic. It was no surprise that the title became his—as the rounds progressed he became stronger and more confident, while his opponent was gradually worn down.

While basking in the glory the next day, Ross made himself a few promises. First, he decided to continue with some training even when no fights were in the wind. After all, he felt and looked good and it would be a shame to throw that all away. And there was no trouble in keeping to his new dietary principles as a year-round plan. There was room and the excuse for a few celebratory meals for the next couple of days, and he could afford to increase his total kilojoule intake now that he was down to his target weight. But gone forever was the on-again, off-again feasting and fasting approach that had been part of his earlier career. He felt on top of the world, and he had the title to prove it!

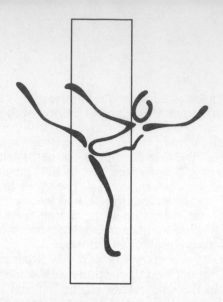

# Gymnastics and diving

Artistic gymnastics and diving are highly skilled sports in which performance is evaluated subjectively by a panel of judges. There are six events in an Olympic men's gymnastic program—floor, pommel horse, rings, vault, parallel bars and the high bar—while the women's program features four events—floor, vault, asymmetric bars and the beam. In each of these disciplines there are compulsory routines, set every four years on an Olympic cycle, as well as optional routines selected by the athlete. There are separate titles for team competition and for individual performers, with the individual prizes being awarded for each event as well as the overall score.

All events in artistic gymnastics are anaerobic in nature, the longest being the floor (about a minute) and the shortest the vault (a few seconds including the approach run). Skill, muscular strength and power relative to body weight are important components of success.

Diving is separated into springboard (1 and 3metre) and highboard (3, 5, 7.5 and 10metre) events for men and women. There are a set number of compulsory and voluntary dives which each competitor must perform. Each dive is marked separately. Numerous combinations of starting position, flight movements and twists differentiate the degree of difficulty of each dive. As in gymnastics, depletion of fuel stores is not a contributing factor to diving performance, with skill and power being the important determinants of success.

Male athletes peak at a much later age than females in these sports. While most top male divers and gymnasts fit within the 18–28 year age range, elite female competitors are much younger. In fact, rules are now in place to restrict females under fourteen years of age from competing in international level gymnastics or platform diving.

## Training

The development of gymnastic skills takes years of intense practice and requires gymnasts to totally commit their lifestyle to the sport. Training begins at an early age, and even by nine or ten years gymnasts in elite development programs may be committed to a training load in excess of twenty hours per week. These programs now begin to prepare athletes four to six years in advance of specific competitions, gradually building up to a full training load of 30–40 hours per week. Typically, eleven or twelve training sessions are undertaken each week, with daily training sessions before and after school or work lasting two or more hours each.

The training load of an elite diver can be equally demanding, with three to four hours per day spent on water work, and another hour of dry-land training. Training generally starts at an early age, reflecting the years of skill and strength development that are required. Occasionally, elite divers emerge from a gymnastics background, changing to diving at a later age after injury or lack of success halt their gymnastics career.

In the non-competitive season, or in the early development of the gymnast or diver, much of the training time is spent on acquiring skills through technique work and body conditioning. Supplementary weight training is often undertaken, particularly by male athletes, and may make up to 25 percent of total training time.

As the athlete matures or as the competitive season draws closer, progressively more time is spent on the development of the compulsory and optional gymnastic routines or dives.

## Competition

There are four separate components in a gymnastics program:

1 Set/compulsory routines on each of the apparatus.
2 Optional routines on each of the apparatus.
3 Individual combined finals, where only the optional routines are performed again.
4 Individual apparatus finals, where the top performers on each apparatus compete again.

This program is spread over four days, with the duration of competition being about two hours per day for each competitor as they rotate between apparatus. A warm-up of a similar length is usually completed before the start of competition, and between performances (from five to 30 minutes apart) competitors may perform stretching exercises.

In diving contests, preliminary rounds are held when there are more than sixteen competitors, and the top twelve competitors proceed to a final. Preliminary rounds may be held on the morning and finals in the evening of the same day. Men perform eleven dives and women, ten dives in springboard events, and in highboard events ten and eight dives are performed respectively. Four or five dives in each event are compulsory, with the remainder being dives selected by the athlete. A diving meet can last four to six days with the competition for each board being held on separate days.

## Physical characteristics

Gymnasts are a physically homogeneous group, the characteristics for elite performance being very marked. The skill and agility of gymnastics requires that an athlete should be small and well-muscled, with a low body-fat level. The physical profile of the female gymnast has changed since the 1970s, with champions such as Olga Corbut and Nadia Comanechi turning attention away from mature female physiques to a youthful almost pre-pubescent look.

In addition to the physical advantages of increased mechanical efficiency and power-to-weight ratio, being small and light conveys a more favourable visual image to gymnastic judges.

Divers share similar physical characteristics to gymnasts, with a compact frame and low body-fat level being important both for physical and aesthetic advantages.

**Typical physique (elite gymnasts)**

|  | Male | Female |
| --- | --- | --- |
| Height | 160–174cm | 154–162cm |
| Weight | 56–70kg | 43–51kg |
| Skinfold sum | 31–47mm | 37–51mm |

## Common nutrition issues

*Body fat and size—are goals realistic?*

Athletes in aesthetically-judged skill sports—gymnastics, diving, figure skating, ballet dancing etc.—are set strict guidelines about weight and skinfold levels. Females, especially, face an uphill battle to achieve or maintain the sparrow-like dimensions that are expected of them. They may have to combat the fat deposition that accompanies puberty, as well as to achieve body-fat goals that are more applicable to endurance training athletes. Although these athletes spend many hours in training each week (or each day), the training load is focused on skill and technique rather than kilojoule-burning aerobic exercise.

The secret of body-fat loss is explained in Chapter 3 and involves increasing the amount of aerobic exercise and/or decreasing food energy intake. When athletes are already training many hours each day, there may be no time for extra aerobic exercise, or the coach may be reluctant to allow an extra training load with a high risk of injury. This leaves the athlete with only one choice—to resort to a low-kilojoule intake. Even with a well-chosen meal plan there may be difficulties to be faced—from inadequate intake of some nutrients to depression of metabolic rate and increased energy efficiency. In some cases the athlete may actually be in a state of chronic low-grade starvation. And this is the best-case scenario. Many athletes enter the cycle of fad diets, disordered eating and eating disorders as they aim to meet their body-fat goals. The disadvantages are then those of undernutrition as well as the side effects of the weight-loss methods used.

For males the problem is not so critical. Males are more likely to naturally arrive at low body-fat levels associated with these sports. However, some will face similar challenges to their female training partners.

Regardless of the sex, it is important that realistic weight and body-fat targets be set for these athletes. While low body-fat levels confer a physical advantage to skill, there is nevertheless also a component of aesthetic value and peer-pressure involved. Why should extremely thin or pre-pubescent athletes be judged as better performers, simply because of their appearance? Above all the health and happiness of the athlete should be taken into account when setting body-fat goals. See Chapter 3 for more details.

*The nutritional needs of adolescence*

Gymnastics and diving begin at an early age, following athletes through late childhood, adolescence, and—if they survive—into adulthood. Growth and puberty exert special nutritional demands, including increased needs for energy and protein for growth, and iron and calcium for the building of bones and blood supply. Where a chronic low-energy intake exists, there is the possibility of nutritional deficiencies and delayed growth and maturity.

A recent study of the physical characteristics of junior elite female gymnasts reported that those in the 7–10 year age group were of average height and weight for their age (around the 50th percentile), but that the 11–14 year olds had slipped back to the 20th percentile in these measures. Muscle mass was high but body fat levels were below average in these groups. The drop in height and weight could indicate:

- that nutritional deficits exist, causing a delay in puberty and growth failure;
- that sports-specific factors are selecting the gymnasts—that is, that the smaller and lighter gymnasts are progressing while heavier and bigger gymnasts drop out of the program; or
- that both factors are operating.

Obviously, there is a need to follow the same group of gymnasts right though to determine which factor is most important. However, a warning is sounded that young gymnasts are nutritionally vulnerable, and that health and growth may be compromised if dietary intake is restricted. It is hoped that gymnastics programs are not so dogmatic that they consciously 'bonsai' their young athletes—that is, consciously restrict their growth by keeping them undernourished. Poor growth patterns are associated with greater disease morbidity, including impaired bone development.

### Amenorrhea and bone impairment

Athletic groups with low body-fat levels, particularly those that seem artificially contrived, may be at an increased risk of amenorrhea. Amenorrhea may be in the form of a failure to start periods altogether, or the cessation of an already established menstrual cycle. A complication of this condition is reduced bone density, and perhaps an increased risk of stress fractures now, and osteoporosis later. Although this problem is worsened by poor calcium intake, it is fundamentally a problem of low estrogen levels, and should be investigated and treated. Read the story of Sharon in the distance running chapter, and see Chapter 2.6 for hints about a good calcium intake.

### Training nutrition—an overview

It has already been established that many gymnasts and divers are at risk of inadequate nutrition, because of their restricted energy intake. Indeed dietary surveys of female gymnasts have reported inadequate intakes of many vitamins and minerals. Read Chapters 1 and 2 for an overview of the nutritional goals of an athlete in heavy training.

Another factor that greatly influences the eating habits of these athletes, is the great time commitment involved in their sport. With the day divided between school, training, homework and, later on a job, there is often little time for cooking and preparing meals—for the athlete or their family. The only people busier than young gymnasts are their mothers—driving them to and from their training, and struggling to meet the needs of all the family members. Meals are often eaten in the car on the way to school, or on the way home from training, and Mum must be creative to organise food that is nutritious, transportable and easily eaten.

## Competition nutrition

Athletes need a meal plan that will fit in with their competition sched-ule, often spread over a number of days. Competition is not likely to threaten fluid and fuel stores, since it is quite brief and low in intensity. However, each athlete needs to find a plan that sits comfortably—both in the stomach and with their confidence. There is no need to carbo-load or undertake severe dietary preparation for an event. Read Chapter 4.2 about general preparation for competition, and Chapter 4.4 for ideas about pre-event meals.

## Eating disorders

With so much pressure to be light and low in body fat, it is not surprising that much of the life, the conversation and the hobbies of female gymnasts and divers revolve around food and weight loss. There is constant attention to what the athlete looks like, how much she weighs or how large her skinfold sum is, all of which are reinforced by other athletes, and often unfortunately, by coaches and parents.

In this environment it is not surprising that eating disorders and disordered eating become apparent amongst female athletes. How else can unrealistic goals be met? And how do you resist when everyone else is doing it? Read the account below to see how the problem covers a spectrum from shared weight-loss activities to desperate and pathological disturbances in eating behaviour. The hazards and the treatment will vary accordingly, but budget for great patience and support and the input of various professionals. The problem also occurs with male athletes but there is a much lower incidence.

PROFILE: CAROL
*Starving for success?*

When Carol took up her new position as head gymnastics coach at the college, she immediately consulted a sports dietitian. She explained that her last job had caused her some unhappiness because of suspected eating disorders amongst some of the female gymnasts. In a new setting and with new students she wanted to tackle the issue with a fresh mind. What could be done to prevent the problem? Was there anything that she did to cause or provoke the situation? How could she detect which girls were having problems and what did she do if difficulties were found?

The dietitian summarised the symptoms of the two major eating disorders, anorexia nervosa and bulimia. While anorexics deny themselves food and generally lose large amounts of body weight, the major feature of bulimia is uncontrolled eating followed by purging, through vomiting or laxative use. In the case of the bulimic, great swings in body weight can be seen. While the syndromes can exist separately, many sufferers show both symptoms, either simultaneously or in tandem. In all cases, there are very clear psychological problems—including disorders in body image and in feelings about food.

The dietitian then explained that eating disorders are not always clearcut. Not every athlete who skips a meal is anorexic, and not everyone who induces vomiting on one occasion is a true bulimic. Instead, there is a spectrum of eating behaviour problems amongst athletes.

At one end of the spectrum are people who suffer with anorexia or bulimia as a primary disorder—that is, a classical psychological disturbance with nutritional consequences. What causes these disorders is unknown, but the symptoms are well recognised and the health implications can be serious. Death is the most extreme outcome—from starvation in the case of the anorexic, from severe electrolyte disturbances in the case of the bulimic, and from suicide in the case of related depression. These disorders also occur in the community, and their numbers include some athletes who then bring the nutritional implications into the sports arena. Extensive treatment is required for both these eating disorders, involving specialised counselling from both psychologists and dietitians, and exploration of interpersonal relationships.

At the other end of the spectrum are athletes with 'occupational' eating disorders—those who have problems with their eating behaviour because they are under pressure to achieve unrealistic nutritional or sporting goals. Achieving or maintaining a low body-fat level is the most common issue, and disordered eating may be expected more commonly amongst athletes or sports that emphasise low body-fat levels. Having been set an unrealistic target of too much or too soon, many athletes turn to bizarre diets, vomiting, laxative use or other problem practices. The other factor that supports the behaviour is peer acceptance. In some sports, body-fat phobia is almost institutionalised, with athletes swapping ideas about weight-loss techniques and making problem eating behaviours seem normal by the virtue of 'everybody' doing it.

The difference between this disordered eating and eating *disorders* is the focus. For the true anorexic, starvation is the end, while for an athlete with an eating behaviour problem, it is the means to the end. In many cases, the athlete when removed from the pressure or the

## SIGNS OF EATING DISORDERS

| | |
|---|---|
| Weight changes | sudden loss of weight<br>wide fluctuations in weight over a short time |
| Food behaviour | consumption of large amounts of food that are inconsistent with the athlete's weight<br>evidence of eating in private (food wrappers or food disappearing etc.)<br>avoidance of eating or refusal to join in social occasions involving eating<br>excessive interest in handling food and in preparing food for others |
| Self-image | worry about being too fat<br>constant self-examination and comparison with others |
| Personality | withdrawn, anxious<br>mood swings |
| Evidence of problem behaviours | admission or evidence that athlete uses diuretics, laxatives or diet pills<br>admisision or evidence that the athlete vomits after meals<br>excessive exercise often in addition to set training program |
| Physical signs | amenorrhea<br>tooth decay/acid erosion of teeth from vomiting<br>stress fractures<br>cold intolerance<br>jaundiced skin (carotenemia)<br>lanugo (fine hair on body) |

environment that condones the behaviour will revert to better eating practices and the problem will disappear. Others, however, may get caught up in a powerfully-sustained cycle and become enmeshed in a true eating disorder.

After listening to this explanation, Carol thought back to her gymnastics career and the memories of her own weight obsession returned. She agreed with the dietitian that the environment had certainly supported disordered eating practices. Having been set unreasonable body-fat targets—by herself, her coach or the sport—she had become driven with the desire to be lean.

'We all thought about food all the time,' she said, 'We weighed ourselves a thousand times a day, and looked at our tummies every time a mirror or shiny surface was passed. The only time I stopped thinking about my next meal, how many Calories, and how much exercise I'd have to do to burn it up, was when I started thinking about my friend and whether she was thinner than I was.

'We were certainly very miserable, although at the time I didn't know any different. We were always trying the latest diet, and one day we bought some diet pills, though they were short-lived and didn't seem to make any difference. Some of my friends could make themselves sick, but I was too frightened to try, in case my mother found out. One girl in the class eventually ended up in hospital after taking too many laxatives, and that gave us all a scare.

'Funnily, I never considered I had a problem, and in fact when I stopped competing in gymnastics I stopped worrying so much. I still like to keep myself in trim, but it's not like the consuming passion that it used to be.'

The dietitian agreed that this was part of the range of eating behaviour problems, and that at any level the athlete experienced disadvantages to physical and emotional health, and to athletic performance. Even if it does not become a life-threatening condition, many athletes worry too much about their food and their body-fat scores. While definite causes of disordered eating and eating disorders can often not be pinpointed or eradicated, it is important to recognise the contribution of both a perfectionist personality on the part of the athlete, and a pressurised environment created by coaches, parents and other athletes.

MAUREEN
*A vegetarian adventure*

When Maureen's older sister came back from a year overseas as an exchange student, she announced to her parents that she had decided to become a vegetarian. One of her foster families had been Seventh Day Adventists, and she had enjoyed their vegetarian lifestyle. After becoming involved with an ecological interest group at her new school she decided that she was ready to take a personal stand on the killing of animals.

Maureen, a state-level diver, was enthusiastic to join the cause. Over the past six months she had become very picky with her food, and the family mealtime had become a bit of a battleground. She explained that being vegetarian would help her keep her skinfolds down, 'I'll never get to the top being this fat,' she said.

The response from other people was less favourable. Maureen's father was aghast at the thought of eating 'hippy food' and warned her that she would be unable to keep up her strength for twenty hours of training a week, let alone her school work. Her diving coach

## HINTS FOR DEALING WITH EATING DISORDERS—
for coaches, training partners and parents

- Recognise athletes with compulsive and perfectionist personalities. While self-drive and motivation are good characteristics for success, many athletes would benefit from counselling in skills of goal setting and achievement rather than behaving as their own worst enemies.

- Create an environment that supports healthy nutrition and weight control principles. Allow athletes to set realistic body weight and body-fat targets, and make healthy nutrition advice accessible— both at a group and individual level.

- Be aware of early signs of disordered eating behaviour (see table on previous page). Recognise that you may be over-reacting, and try to be objective in collecting evidence of a suspected problem.

- If appropriate, confront the athlete carefully. Express concern, and talk only about objective data—changes in performance, signs of unhappiness, etc. Do not label the athlete or try to diagnose. The athlete may attempt to deny the problem, so stick to discussing hard evidence.

- If it is not appropriate for you to talk to the athlete, speak to someone who can—perhaps the coach or the team doctor, or someone in the athlete's family.

- Seek professional help. It is not your problem—and you are not trained to deal with it. You may have the consent of the athlete to organise this step. Alternatively you may have to wait for the right moment before the help is accepted. Sometimes you may need to withdraw your support of the athlete until this step is taken. Make sure that they are clear that you still care for them, but you do not support their behaviour.

  Professional assessment and counselling should probably involve both a psychologist and a dietitian—make sure that you know of services that specialise in this field.

- Support the professional advice and treatment plan. Try not to become embroiled in the problem, but remain caring, supportive and objective. Be prepared to be patient and flexible—the athlete may need constant reassessment of their goals.

was also tentative—the only vegetarian athlete he had trained had become anemic and dropped out of competition. Finally her mother mediated in the dispute and took Maureen to see a sports dietitian. She had two questions:

1   Is a vegetarian diet healthy? and
2   Can a successful athlete be a vegetarian?

At the world level, there are millions of people who eat vegetarian diets, and for many cultures and populations this is the normal way of life. By contrast, in Australia, it is more often an individual choice rather than an organised eating pattern.

People choose to be vegetarians for a variety of reasons—because of cultural or religious backgrounds, due to moral or ecological beliefs, because of food availability or financial considerations, because they think it is healthy, and sometimes, simply because it is trendy.

Whatever the reasons, the advantages and disadvantages of vegetarian eating are not clear-cut. Vegetarianism is used to cover a wide variety of food patterns which may have quite different outcomes on health and athletic performance. To most people, being a vegetarian simply means not eating meat, but this is a gross simplification of the total dietary plan. In fact there are many levels of vegetarian eating, including:

- lacto-ovo-vegetarians who eliminate meat, fish and poultry, but who eat dairy products and eggs;
- vegans who eliminate all animal products; and
- part-time vegetarians, who rely on vegetarian meals most of the time but freely depart from this pattern, particularly on social occasions.

The best examples of vegetarian eating are seen in communities or established groups which have practised it for generations, such as Seventh Day Adventists, certain religious orders and the Hare Krishna sect. These people have developed alternative eating patterns and food uses to replace the animal foods that we normally eat. Extensive use is made of nuts, seeds and legumes (beans and pulses), and a greater variety of cereals, fruits and vegetables is explored. Many food products, for example, can be derived from soya beans, including soya milk and tofu curd.

Recipes, clever food combinations, and other healthy nutrition secrets are passed between members of the vegetarian community, and the food supply is usually geared to make a variety of vegetarian foods available and cheap. Amongst such well organised groups it is rare to see nutritional deficiencies, since their food patterns have been been carefully thought out and developed over long periods of time. The emphasis is not on what they are giving up but on how they can enjoy a wider variety of other (vegetable) foods to supply their nutritional requirements.

Compare this with a modern vegetarian who thinks that the message is simply to give up meat. In the worst-case scenario, we see people

sitting down to a pile of steamed vegetables minus the traditional lamb-chop, or pulling the ham out of their ham sandwich and thinking that this is a healthy way to eat. Many 'nouveau-vegetarians' make no attempt to replace the nutrients that have been eliminated along with the foods they have given up. Maybe they are too busy feeling virtuous from the thought of giving up fat and chemicals (or the other 'nasties' they think are in animal foods). Maybe they do not know how to explore the world of grains and legumes, and their cooking skills are limited. Or, maybe these new food supplies are hard to get and expensive, because they are going against the tide of the general community eating patterns.

How healthy a vegetarian diet is depends on the individual vegetarian. When vegetarian eating is planned and adventurous, it has the promise of being low in fat and salt, and high in carbohydrate and fibre. This should sound familiar, as it is the blue-print for healthy eating and the optimum training diet for an athlete.

Studies of established vegetarian communities generally show lower rates of heart disease, obesity and high blood pressure than seen in meat-eating Western groups. Of course, these problems are not entirely the result of eating animal foods per se, but from the tendency of the modern Western diet to be high in fat and salt, and low in fibre and carbohydrate. The Western diet can be modified to turn around this profile without removing all animal foods. The important point is that a well-planned vegetarian diet can be as healthy as a well-planned meat-containing diet, but that badly-planned diets of both types are unlikely to fulfil the nutritional goals for health and athletic performance.

What are the traps of a hit-and-miss vegetarian diet? Firstly, there are the problems of inadequate nutrient intake, and of eating insufficient kilojoules because of the bulkiness of plant foods. Eliminating animal foods leaves a vacuum in terms of protein (meats, eggs and dairy products), iron, zinc and other trace elements (especially red meats and shellfish) and calcium (dairy products). Finding suitable replacements from vegetable foods is sometimes tricky, since the vegetable food source may be lower in nutrient content, and the availability of the nutrient (how well your body can absorb and use the nutrient) may be lower than in the animal food form. This is true for protein (read Chapter 2.3 about mixing and matching vegetable proteins to improve their amino acid profile) and for iron (read Chapter 2.5 about making vegetable iron sources available to the body). Occasionally other nutrients, such as some of the B-vitamins, fall into short supply in a restricted vegetarian diet.

In general, the risks of nutrient deficiencies are greater for those who have increased dietary requirements and for those who restrict their food range to the greatest extent. Into the former category go females (iron), adolescents (protein, energy, iron and calcium) and heavily training athletes, while the latter group includes vegans and the unimaginative vegetarian eaters mentioned already.

## SPECIAL ISSUES IN VEGETARIAN EATING

| Nutritional issue | Sources | Comments |
|---|---|---|
| Variety | all foods | Choose to be lacto-ovo-vegetarian (eating eggs and dairy products) rather than vegan, *or* enjoy a range of both vegetarian and meat-based meals—the more variety the better. |
| Energy (kilojoules) | all food | To keep up a high kilojoule intake:<br>— spread food into six or seven meals, rather than three large ones<br>— make high-energy drinks such as fruit smoothies or make use of liquid meal supplements<br>— avoid excessive fibre intake, and include some less bulky refined carbohydrate foods such as juices, white bread and white pastas (see Chapter 3.7).<br><br>To avoid excess kilojoule intake:<br>— watch the total quantity that you eat (healthy doesn't necessarily mean low-joule)<br>— limit intake of fats and oils. |
| Fats and oils | oils<br>margarine<br>cheese<br>pastry<br>nuts & seeds<br>cream | Limit fat and oil in cooking, and vegetarian recipes based on pastry, cream and cheese (see Chapter 1.2 for general ideas). |
| Carbohydrate | grains<br>cereals<br>fruits<br>starchy vegies<br>legumes<br>flavoured<br>  low-fat dairy<br>  foods | This is your chance to try new foods and learn different ways of cooking. Make nutritious carbohydrate foods your first choice—they will also be an important source of protein vitamins and minerals. |

| Nutritional issue | Sources | Comments |
|---|---|---|
| Protein | low-fat dairy foods<br>eggs<br>legumes<br>nuts & seeds<br>wholegrains & cereals<br>soy products<br>liquid meal supplements | The quality of vegetable protein can be improved by mixing with a small amount of animal protein (dairy food or eggs) or by matching with another vegetable food. Good matches are cereals/grains and legumes, or legumes and nuts/seeds (see Chapter 2.3). |
| Iron | wholegrain cereals—esp. breakfast cereal<br>legumes<br>nuts & seeds<br>tofu & soy products<br>eggs<br>green leafy vegies<br>dried fruit<br>liquid meal supplements | Add a vitamin C food to the meal to increase the iron absorption, avoid excessive fibre intake (see Chapter 2.5). |
| Zinc and trace minerals | eggs<br>other iron-rich foods | Generally, if you look after iron intake, other minerals will also be looked after. |

The other problem, especially in the case of new players, is that vegetarian food is not necessarily healthy. While plant foods are generally carbohydrate-based, heavy use of vegetable oils in cooking, high-fat pastries and batters on food, and the addition of cream and cheese to recipes, all produce a high-kilojoule, high-fat meal. Some vegetarians, while refusing meat because they believe that it is high in fat, will continue to use full-cream dairy products and to cook with high-fat methods. Clearly, such a diet will not achieve the health and performance advantages that they seek. In fact, some new 'vegos' actually gain weight with this high-fat intake and end up worse off than before.

So, vegetarianism: to be or not to be? For moral, religious or cultural reasons the choice may be clear cut, and athlete or not, such a decision should be respected. Maureen's sister fits into this category, and in making the choice to be vegetarian she must also accept certain responsibilities. It may be harder for her to meet her nutritional needs, especially living amongst a meat-eating community, and she will need to be organised to make this happen. The table below presents a summary of some of the issues of vegetarian eating.

From the health or athletic performance perspective, the choice doesn't need be so black and white. There are both nutritional advantages and disadvantages to vegetarian eating, but the best of both worlds can be easily achieved—as Maureen found out. With the blessing of her parents and the help of her sister, she has started to explore the world of vegetarian food. Twice a week, they experiment with different recipes, from vegetable and tofu stir-fries and lentil burgers, to bean sauces for pasta.

Learning about these foods has helped her understand more about nutrition in general, and on the nights that she eats meat, fish and chicken meals she uses some of the ideas from her vegetarian cook books to add plenty of carbohydrate foods and cut down the fats. Not only has she begun to enjoy food and nutrition, but her skinfold problem has slowly started to look after itself, with much less panic than before.

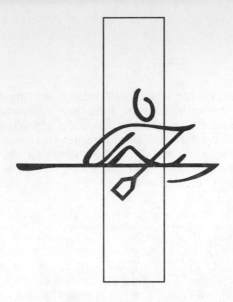

# Rowing

In international competition, both male and female crews race over a distance of 2000 metres. Crews are distinguished by the number of members in the boat (singles, doubles, fours and eights), whether there is a coxswain steering (the pairs and quads may be coxed or coxless), and whether the boat is sculled (two oars per person) or rowed (one oar each).

In some competitions, there is a separate lightweight division in which male rowers or scullers are not permitted to exceed 72.5kg with a crew average of 70kg, and in which the weight limits for women are 59kg (maximum) and 57kg (crew average). Although lightweight competition has been trialled at World Rowing Championship level, only the open or heavyweight competition is conducted at the Olympic Games.

Weight limits also exist for the coxes, being 50kg for males and 40kg for women.

At elite levels, the time taken to complete the 2000-metre race ranges from over seven minutes for the singles to around 5.5 minutes for the eights. Since both arms and legs are active, representing a large proportion of total body muscle mass, considerable cardiovascular and metabolic demands are made. Rowing places great demands on both the aerobic and anaerobic energy systems, with the mean oxygen consumption for a race being not far short of the maximum achievable.

## Training

Rowing training is long and intense. For eight to ten months of the year, rowing training consists of about twelve sessions per week, with nine on the water and three in the gymnasium. At times some crews make an even greater commitment, with two water sessions and a gym session in the one day. A typical rowing session covers about twenty kilometres at a heart rate high enough to stress both aerobic and anaerobic (lactic) metabolism. Weight training sessions are undertaken to improve muscular endurance.

## Competition

Depending on the stature of the regatta, competition may last from three days to a week. Scullers and crews are first drawn in heats, with successful competitors progressing to semi-finals or finals, and the remainder to a repechage. Competitors successful in the repechage may progress to a semi-final. In large competitions, rowers will be required to race only once per day, however they may be required to race as hard on the first day as in the finals, to keep progressing through the competition. Light training is undertaken on rest days.

In lightweight competition, weigh-ins are conducted on the mornings of the events.

## Physical characteristics

Heavyweight rowers are tall and heavy, with strong muscles and long limbs being favourable characteristics. Since the load is held constant (weight limits for the boat and coxswain), a larger and heavier crew has an advantage over a physically smaller crew. While muscle mass should account for most of the athlete's increased weight, body-fat levels are often relatively high among heavy-weight rowers, particularly females.

Lightweight crews are obviously smaller and lighter than their heavyweight counterparts, with lower body-fat levels showing the importance of a high power-to-weight ratio. As in most sports with weight divisions, many athletes 'sit on the fence' of the weight limits—being too small and light to compete successfully against bigger and stronger athletes, but nevertheless struggling to fit naturally into the lower weight limit.

**Typical physique (elite heavyweight rowers)**

|  | Male | Female |
| --- | --- | --- |
| Height | 187–195cm | 174–181cm |
| Weight | 87–93kg | 65–76kg |
| Skinfold sum | 38–56mm | 72–114mm |

## Common nutrition issues

### Training nutrition—high energy and carbohydrate requirements

Rowers can face enormous energy and carbohydrate requirements to support their heavy training loads and body weight/strength goals. Males especially fight to keep their body weight up while all rowers must work hard to recover from one day to the next. The lifestyle of the rower can also interfere with meeting these huge requirements. The time spent at training is time that isn't spent eating, and as in the case of Terry below, many rowers find it difficult to chew and stomach the amounts of food they need in a day.

Read Chapters 1 and 2 for details of the optimum training diet. A high-energy, high-carbohydrate, highly nutritious diet should be on the menu to achieve all the goals of heavy training. A pattern of small frequent meals, including a carbohydrate snack immediately after training, is the best plan of attack—allowing high energy goals to be achieved (Chapter 3.7) and recovery to be maximised (Chapter 5). Of course, this means being organised—see the case of Terry below.

### Matters of physique

Higher body-fat levels are not as great a disadvantage to a rower as they are to a distance runner. After all, it is an advantage to be heavy and strong, and body weight is supported in the boat. However, there is a limit to the excess baggage that can be carried. It is better to be 80kg with body fat of 50mm, rather than 80kg with a body fat of 100mm. Lightweight crews have a definite need to optimise their power-to-weight ratio.

At some stage you may need to undertake special programs either to gain lean body mass or lose body fat. See Chapter 3 for advice.

### Females and iron status

Female rowers face the risk of poor iron status, reflecting both their sex and their training commitment. Read Chapter 2.5 for advice about a high-iron diet that is also high in carbohydrate. Regular checks of iron status are recommended, especially where a previous history of iron deficiency exists. Male rowers may also need to be aware of possible problems with iron, particularly during adolescence when iron requirements are increased to cover growth costs.

### Fluid needs

Long training sessions on the water in hot weather lead to significant sweat losses, particularly when undertaken twice a day. Learn good hydration practices in training—drink before sessions, take a water bottle to training, and rehydrate fully afterwards. Weighing yourself before and after training sessions for a week will give you a clear picture of your body's fluid swings. You may like to use a sports drink during and after long training sessions—experiment to see if your training performance is improved.

## Competition nutrition

Rowers should go into each race with fluid and fuel stores topped up, and feeling comfortable after the last meal. With the regatta or competition lasting a number of days, the challenge is set to recover between each day's sessions and to repeat these goals for the next race.

Read Chapter 4 for advice about competition nutrition, and Chapter 5 for strategies to promote rapid recovery. Special care may be needed with pre-event eating—it can be very uncomfortable to race with a full stomach. Liquid meals may come in handy as a low-bulk pre-event meal or snack. With much of the day tied up in preparation and the race itself, there is usually neither time nor opportunity for rowers to meet their usual high-energy intake. Consequently, some rowers find that they quickly lose weight over the course of the competition.

Whether it be for an energy boost, or for a well-timed post-race recovery snack, it makes good sense for rowers to have nutritious food supplies at their finger-tips at all times. This might mean organising suitable supplies both at the rowing site and at the competition accommodation. Don't rely on the event organisers to have thought of your needs. Liquid meal supplements are again useful, being low in bulk, nutritious and portable. Use your creativity to think up other snacks as well.

Finally, don't neglect fluid needs. You may be dehydrated through your effort, through your making-weight practices (see below), or just from sitting out in the sun watching the rest of the competition. Carbohydrate-containing fluids such as sports drinks can be useful for both fluid and carbohydrate top-ups.

## Lightweight rowing

As in other weight-matched sports, many rowers attempt to row in lightweight competition when their training weight is well above the event limits. For many lightweight rowers, obsession with food and weight, leading to disordered eating and eating disorders, becomes part of the way of life. This is topped off with severe dehydration and food restriction in the days leading up to competition—practices which may be repeated over the duration of the rowing competition. Females seem to be most at risk, although these problems are also experienced in male crews.

There is no doubt that these measures are harmful—physically and mentally—and affect both health and performance. From the performance perspective, a rowing competition is an extremely severe exercise challenge that should not be attempted at less than optimum preparation. The long-term consequences of a rowing career include the potential for disturbed metabolic efficiency. It is not unusual to find rowers complaining of increased difficulty in losing weight as time progresses, eventually reaching the point that, even with heavy training and sparrow-like intakes, they seem to be in energy balance. There are many additional disadvantages to health and nutritional status.

Read Chapter 3, and the account of Maree below for alternative ways to deal with the issue. Commonsense is often overlooked because crazy weight control practices become entrenched in the sport. Unfortunately, they can even be glorified. From the commentary box during the 1990 World Rowing Championships came the following encouragement 'And let's give a big hand to the crew from X—these girls have not eaten anything for four days to make it into this final. What a heroic effort'.

*The life of the cox*

The coxswain's life is not easy. There is usually the pressure of making weight (the crew obviously wants the cox to be as light as possible), as well as the responsibility of keeping the crew together in stroke and spirit. It takes a distinctive sort of personality to rule over the boat. Weight control is made a little more difficult for coxes given that their job is not energy-burning—they are more or less there for the ride.

Since a cox may be involved in many hours of other people's training each day, there is often little time or incentive to take on additional aerobic exercise to aid their own weight control goals. This puts more pressure on reduced energy intake to reduce body-fat levels. Many get caught up in the vicious cycle of making weight through dehydration and starvation, and in a general obsessiveness about food and weight. As in other sports this will have a detrimental effect on health, and like the lightweight rowers, an energy efficiency may develop, making the weight situation worse.

The issues of making weight have been dealt with for lightweight rowers, and in the wrestling and boxing chapter. The same advice is repeated below, and can be followed up in more detail in Chapter 3:

- make sensible decisions about weight targets;
- try to achieve body-fat loss though healthy nutrition and exercise plans, even if that means additional aerobic training; and
- avoid severe dehydration and food restriction practices before competitions.

If you won't do it for yourself, do it for the team. The last thing a top crew needs to face before important competition is an irritable and fatigued cox!

PROFILE: TERRY
*Fitting enough food into the day—and into your stomach*

Terry was living in a university college and rowing with the university coxed fours. The training schedule leading into the competition season was intense—ten water sessions and three weight training sessions each week. The energy requirements were obviously enormous, because Terry was fighting a losing battle to maintain his weight. Not only was he becoming tired, but he was starting to give away over five kilograms on the average crew weight. He was careful to eat a high carbohydrate diet. He had learned all about that in the nutrition classes of his physical education degree at university. But where he could find the time, the stomach room and food to increase his intake, he didn't know. He was already suffering from heartburn, especially when he bent over the oars, and on a couple of occasions he had actually vomited. Naturally, he was reluctant to increase his meal size any further.

He sought help from a sports dietitian after the third consecutive drop in his skinfold readings. She took a detailed account of his typical daily training and eating habits, as summarised below.

The dietitian was pleased with Terry's level of nutrition knowledge. He had a good understanding of carbohydrate foods and was able to make these the focus of all his meals. However, he simply wasn't eating enough, and the dietitian picked out two reasons for this.

- He was limited to eating three times a day, firstly because the university dining hall catered for this, and secondly because his time was tied up between meals. Training took up four or five hours a day, but he was also confined to class or study for a similar time.

- Terry was often caught between eating too little or aggravating his heartburn problems with a huge meal.

The solution lay in making practical changes to increase food opportunities and to change the bulkiness of the meals. Terry was right about the problem of eating too much food at one sitting—however, with a pattern of six or seven meals and snacks a day, and with the clever use of nutritious drinks (low-bulk and high-energy) he could eat a high-energy intake without causing gastrointestinal distress.

Firstly, Terry needed to have increased access to food. The dietitian met with the chef at the university dining hall and negotiated a plan for his special needs. The chef was happy to provide Terry with some food for his room—all rooms were provided with a small fridge and tea-making facilities. Terry would receive some supplies of break-

**A day in the life of Terry (rower)**

| | |
|---|---|
| 5.30–8.00am | Rowing at river<br>Often has heartburn from too much food the previous evening. |
| 8.30am | Back to university college for as much breakfast as can be scoffed in 25 minutes:<br>Cereal + tinned fruit + milk<br>Fruit juice<br>Toast + baked beans or spaghetti |
| 9.15–12.30pm | University classes<br>Indigestion and heartburn |
| 12.45pm | Lunch at University cafeteria<br>(Packed lunch provided by university college):<br>Sandwiches/rolls with meat and salad fillings<br>Fruit bun<br>Fruit juice<br>Sometimes has to cut back the amount if heartburn is bad—can't risk too much discomfort for evening session |
| 1.45–4.30pm | University classes |
| 5.00–7.30pm | Training at river<br>Weights sessions 3/week following rowing |
| 8.00pm | Early nights—arrives at the university dining hall just in time for late meal sitting:<br>Meat/fish/chicken—large serves (often 2 meals)<br>Rice or potatoes—sometimes pasta<br>Vegies or salad<br>Bread<br>Jelly/fruit salad/rice pudding/icecream |
| | Late nights—misses the official meal time.<br>Makes jam sandwiches—sometimes almost a loaf of bread.<br>Probably eats too much, but what else can he do? |
| 9.00–10.30pm | Study<br>Bed |

fast cereal, milk, canned fruit, and muesli bars. And he was encouraged to order two 'lunch bags' for each day—one to be eaten as a morning tea and lunch, and one to be kept as a snack between rowing and the weight session at night. Sandwiches, buns and fruit were easily eaten in the back of class, so he could divide the one meal bag into two sittings, and avoid the discomfort of a single big lunch.

As for the evening meal, the chef made plans to keep a meal waiting on the nights that he was late. Having already had a snack, this would top up his night intake.

Next item on the agenda was to learn how to make nutritious high-energy drinks. Terry was encouraged to invest in a Bamix to mix up delicious concoctions of Sustagen powder, milk, fruit, and low-fat yoghurt or icecream. He could afford to cut down the size of his dinner and breakfast meals and then boost energy intake with 300–500ml of an action-packed drink. This left him able to have a mid-morning and late-evening snack without feeling sick, and his lunch bag or the supplies in his room filled in this gap.

Exceed Sports Nutrition supplement, a ready-to-go version of his high-energy drink, was purchased for an afternoon snack in class. This left him relatively light and empty for the afternoon training session, yet continued to pour in the fuel. Lastly a sports drink was added, to drink in the boat and as soon as the session was over. While he was rehydrating he might as well pump in a little extra carbohydrate. Being able to consume this straight after training was an added bonus for recovery of muscle glycogen stores.

With consistent practice of this plan, Terry gradually began to regain the kilos and find new vigour at training. The heartburn and bloatedness after meals was also greatly reduced, making him feel better in the boat. It was sometimes a nuisance having to be so organised, and unless he kept varying his drink concoctions he became bored with the same thing three times a day. But while he remained one jump ahead of himself, he remained streets ahead in performance.

PROFILE: MAREE
*Rowing lightweight*

Maree tried out for selection in the state rowing squad as a lightweight single sculler. She did well in the physiological testing, and was assessed as having a good stroke technique. Inevitably the scales poked their way into the assessment, and the news was discouraging. At 63.5kg she was nearly five kilograms over the competition weight limit of 59kg. Some of the other girls were even worse off than this—two were up to nearly 69kg. One of these girls had collapsed in her last race, clearly exhausted and dehydrated, and she had had to go to the medical tent for intravenous rehydration.

Maree's own battle with the scales was gradually becoming a losing struggle. When she started rowing four years ago she hovered around 60–61kg, and needed only a small push in competition week to make the weight limit. At first the whole business had seemed exciting and mystical. She had watched the pairs and fours carrying out the weight-loss rituals as a team, and thought that it would bond their spirit together. Later down the track, though, it had become harder and harder to get the weight off, and she had realised that weeks of starving, and days of sitting in saunas or running in thick tracksuits, made teams irritable and squabbling rather than close and cohesive. The crews were allowed to average their weights, so there was always niggling within the team about who should lose more weight and who was letting the others down.

Maree's weight thoughts were now no longer confined to the week leading up to competition, but had become a full-time obsession. She was constantly trying to shed the kilos, and the more she tried the harder it became. If worry was supposed to make you lose weight, then she shouldn't have a problem. Thoughts of food and the scales filled her every waking hour, but all to no avail. The frustration took any of the former enjoyment out of her sport.

She didn't tell this to the selection coach, but then she didn't need to. The trials and tribulations of lightweight rowing were well known to him. He was well aware of the constant dieting, and of the dangerous techniques of sweating and fasting that occurred in competition. He explained to Maree that he was not prepared to support this system, and was only interested in recruiting girls who could safely and healthily row in the lightweight division. While it might be cruel to turn people away, he did not want to be part of the misery and the damage.

The coach looked at Maree's skinfold levels—a sum of 81mm over seven sites. This was higher than it needed to be, giving Maree a real chance to lose weight. He also took into consideration that she had not yet had a mishap during competition. Maree had always rowed well, and could truthfully say that she had never resorted to the more severe weight loss practices of diuretics, laxatives and vomiting. The final decision was to award Maree a temporary scholarship—to be revised in ten weeks. The conditions were that she would see a sports dietitian, and would reduce her training weight to 60–61kg, with a measurable loss from her skinfold levels.

Maree agreed to this trial, but wondered about the usefulness of seeing a dietitian. She wondered what the dietitian could tell her about weight loss that she didn't already know—Maree felt that she had been there, done that when it came to diets. Nevertheless, she kept to her side of the bargain.

The dietitian listened to Maree's story of constant dieting, and her state of learned metabolic efficiency. She certainly seemed to have depressed her energy requirements through years of restricted kilojoule intake and yo-yo weight loss. Her daily eating patterns were described as follows:

**A day in the life of Maree—lightweight sculler**

| | |
|---|---|
| 6.00–8.00am | Rowing training |
| 8.30am | 2 green apples on the way to work |
| 9.00–12.30pm | Work—numerous cups of black tea |
| 12.30pm | Run at lunch time<br>Salad sandwich—no margarine<br>        no meat or cheese |
| 1.30–4.30pm | More tea at work |
| 5.00–7.30pm | Rowing training and weights |
| 8.00pm | Tea at home:<br>Plate of steamed vegetables<br>1–2/week piece of meat or chicken |
| 9.00pm | Green apple |
| Every couple of days—splurges with a block of chocolate | |

The dietitian assessed the daily plan as low in kilojoules, and inadequate in protein, iron, calcium and other minerals. It was a wonder that she was able to keep up her training load with such a small intake of carbohydrate and energy. She suggested that Maree was probably not always aware of the extent of her splurges—and would be surprised to see how her total energy intake fluctuated.

With a 'nothing else to lose' attitude, Maree agreed to try the dietitian's meal plan which included:

- the minimum level of kilojoule intake that could be regarded as healthy (5000 kilojoules or 1200 Cals per day);
- improved intake of protein, carbohydrate and minerals to support training and health requirements;
- a small treat each week;
- a low-dose broad-range vitamin/mineral tablet each day to ensure that all nutrient RDIs were met;
- foods chosen to fit with portable lifestyle—e.g. a breakfast that can be eaten on the way to work (see summary below).

She warned that Maree's greatest need was to begin to let go of her fears and worries, and to think more positively about her food and weight. With confidence and a happier outlook, she would be less likely to get out of control and splurge. This would need a lot of self-talk and support—after all she would need to reverse years of misery and frustration. She scheduled a weekly appointment for Maree to

**Maree's new eating plan**

| | |
|---|---|
| After training | carton of non-fat fruit yoghurt<br>piece of fruit (change for variety) |
| Lunch | salad sandwich with lean meat/chicken/<br>salmon no margarine<br>water or low-joule drinks<br>small tub of fresh fruit salad |
| Dinner (straight after training) | 100g serve of lean red meat/chicken/fish<br>potato or small serve of rice<br>1 slice bread (no margarine)<br>low-joule drinks |
| Supper | small bowl of breakfast cereal<br>skim milk |
| Twice a week | chocolate frog |
| Analysis: | 5000 kilojoules (1200 Cals)<br>75g of protein<br>200g of carbohydrate (= 62% of energy)<br><br>Iron = 12mg<br>Calcium = 880mg<br><br>Vitamins meet RDI intake and are insured by additional mulitivitamin supplement. |

come and talk about her progress, and promised her that no scales would appear during that time. The emphasis would be on how Maree was feeling and coping.

Progress was slow but sure. Maree needed a lot of encouragement to change her old way of thinking. She agreed that she was happy with the meal plan, but needed to remind herself that a small treat was OK on occasions, and that she didn't need to watch the scales or have all the weight off within a week.

The first weight and skinfold check-in was after a month. The results were encouraging—weight was 62kg and skinfolds were 68mm. At the end of the second month, there was further progress—weight was 61kg and skinfolds 60mm. She met with the coach a fortnight later with a big smile on her face, and weighed in at 60.5kg. With a little fine-tuning before competition, and the nerves that went with big races, she would be well able to meet event limits. The rewards for her effort were not only a full rowing scholarship, but a totally changed outlook on her life and her sport.

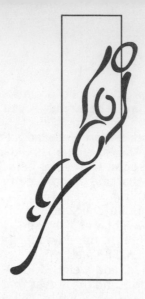

# Australian Rules Football

Australian Rules Football is played predominantly by males, with the major league, the Australian Football League, having developed into a national competition. It is played from primary school upwards, at a variety of levels both amateur and professional.

A game is made up of four 25 minute quarters, with time-on (usually five to ten minutes) added for the time that the ball is out of play. The first and third quarters are separated by a short break, with a longer break at half-time. Each team consists of eighteen players on the ground, with another two 'interchange' players who may be swapped at any time for other players on the field.

The traditional line-up sees five lines of three players spread from one end of the ground (backs) to the other (forwards), with the other three players set to follow the play. However, as the game has evolved into a more mobile style of play, these traditional lines have lost much of their former meaning. In addition to running, players must leap to mark or punch the ball. Heavy physical contact and tackling also increase the demands on players.

## Training

The football year can be divided into three sections: pre-season, season, and off-season. The length of each section will vary with the level of competition. A typical outline might be:

- Off-season: 1–3 months from October–January—little or no scheduled training. Often a time where body fat increases.
- Pre-season: 2–4 months—training may start as early as November with 3 to 5 sessions per week. Individual players are often selected for specific programs according to the requirements of their position or their individual weaknesses. In general, training revolves around a running program, building up an aerobic base and then anaerobic speed and endurance. Weight training is built into the program—especially for players who need to build up bulk and strength. Other sports such as boxing or swimming may also be included. Skills training is introduced as pre-season progresses, with practice matches leading into the season.
- Competitive season: There are roughly six days between matches. Most clubs schedule three or four training sessions between these games, with a heavy session mid-week, and lighter skill-oriented sessions later in the week.

Most training sessions are held in the late afternoon to fit in with work schedules.

## Competition

The AFL season consists of 22 games, one played each weekend from March to August, with finals being held in September. Most games are played on Saturday or Sunday afternoons with the under-age and reserve matches preceding the main game. The national competition now involves interstate travel, with some games being played at night under lights. A supplementary night competition and pre-season practice matches generally start in early February and may add another six matches to the year's tally.

An Australian Rules Football match lasts about two hours, with the physiological demands varying considerably between field positions. On-ball players may run between twelve and twenty kilometres each match, with a fairly even proportion of aerobic and anaerobic activities and a high total-fuel requirement. Typically players run at top speed for 10–50 metres, followed by a walk or jog back to position.

Full-forwards and full-backs perform very short, high-intensity sprints with almost purely anaerobic requirements and lower total energy demands.

The repeated physical contact and the resulting damage to muscle fibres must be taken into consideration in the recovery between matches.

### Physical characteristics

The Australian Rules Football team has been introduced as a mixed bag of field positions and playing skills. It should come as no surprise that the physical profile of the Australian Rules Football player is varied—from 200cm rucks to 170cm rovers. Lower body-fat levels are expected amongst running players. Greater height and muscle mass are expected in key positions where players directly contest each other for the ball.

### Other comments

Tradition has played a strong role in the development of Australian Rules football. Many competition and training practices have persisted long after they have become outdated by scientific thinking—often because players become coaches or trainers and pass on the old methods. Fortunately, accredited courses for coaches and trainers are gradually causing the death of many old wives' tales.

Another characteristic which has helped to retain tradition is the close-knit environment of the team and the persuasive power of peer influence. Attitudes and behaviour are shared, and because 'everybody' does something, it is regarded as normal, even when the practice is not normal outside the football club, or for that matter, a sensible and healthy practice.

Despite this, Australian Rules Football has changed dramatically in the past twenty years and now requires greater commitment and professionalism from players. Today's footballers play a different style of game to that played by their childhood heroes. The new game is faster, and requires players to be fitter both in terms of speed and endurance. Players must also look more closely at recovery—both within and after the game, then through the week's training to the next match. Although there has been some progress in the scientific basis of training and match preparation, there are still many areas that are yet to be refined.

### Common nutrition issues

#### General nutrition knowledge and cooking skills

The top football leagues begin to recruit new players as young as fifteen or sixteen years. This sometimes means relocating young players to a new city. Accommodation is often found with families, however many young recruits and indeed older players share houses in which no-one has any real nutrition knowledge or cooking skills.

Even at the professional level, most footballers have full-time employment. When the heavy commitment of training, matches and other club activities are added to work hours, there may be little time for food shopping and preparation. A pattern of skipped meals and reliance on take-away foods is common.

Australian Rules Football players should be screened to find those at risk. Basic nutrition education and cooking lessons can be a valuable tool in improving the dietary intake of these players.

## Take-aways and restaurants

Take-away foods are typical fare for weekends (after the game) and may become the staple of footballers who can't cook for themselves. Upgraded cooking skills should enable quick and easy meals to be made at home. However, players should also be educated about good choices with take-aways, and how to eat well in restaurants. It is inevitable that these opportunities will continue to contribute to food intake, but with careful selection they should also be able to contribute to total nutrition goals. See the section on takeaways in the Basketball chapter.

## Weight control—or more importantly, control of body fat

Many players start pre-season or come back from injury heavier than their usual playing weight. In football circles, the traditional emphasis has been on total body weight rather than an understanding of muscle mass versus body fat. Ideally, clubs should arrange for someone on their sports medicine/fitness staff to be trained to take skinfold measurements. Body-fat levels should be monitored at strategic times of the football year and individual targets set for each player. Chapter 3 explains how body-fat measurements are taken and how body-fat goals are set. Footballers are notorious for using crash and fad diets to achieve weight loss. For a better approach to steady and permanent loss of body fat, read Chapter 3.3. Rodney's story below shows how this can work in real-life.

## Gaining muscle mass

At the other end of spectrum is the young slightly-built recruit who wishes to gain weight to withstand the physical contact of the game. In actual fact, it is a gain of muscle mass and strength that is required. As outlined in Chapters 3.6 and 3.7, bulking up requires an appropriate weights program, a high-energy diet and realistic expectations. In addition, specialist coaching may help slender players to adopt body-positioning and game skills that overcome many of the problems of being pushed around.

## Alcohol intake

The alcohol intake of many footballers is a good example of the power of peer group behaviour over principles of peak training nutrition—

and even plain commonsense. The typical drinking patterns of Australian Rules Football players are examined in the account at the end of this chapter. Although football players rationalise that this is normal, poor use of alcohol will prevent optimum performance from being reached in a number of ways. A better approach to alcohol in sport is presented in Chapter 1.6.

### Recovery and muscle glycogen

Traditionally, football players have considered carbohydrate only on the eve of the match. The sentiment has been to eat protein at the beginning of the week, carbohydrate at the end. Yet recovery from a match, and between each training session, requires a high carbohydrate intake *every* day. It is likely that the game combined with long training nights will draw heavily on muscle glycogen stores particularly for running players. Muscle damage and injury, caused for example by body contact and tackling, will require even higher carbohydrate intakes to promote glycogen restoration.

Active recovery should begin as soon as each exercise session finishes. The study reported below shows that elite footballers are not aware of this. They eat a typical Australian training diet rather than the high-carbohydrate diet needed to promote muscle glycogen refuelling. And the most crucial period for active recovery—immediately after the game—is probably the time that nutritional needs are most neglected.

Read Chapter 5 on active recovery and then organise your post-match activities to look after fluid and carbohydrate replacement. Perhaps your club can organise a suitable post-match function to encourage this as a team priority. Daily recovery of fuel stores will require a high carbohydrate intake all week round, starting straight after each training session. Read Chapters 1.3 and 2.2 for hints on everyday use of carbohydrate foods. The ability to bounce back immediately from each match and training session should give you edge over your opponents, and save you from that end-of-the-week fatigue.

### Preparation for the match

When footballers started thinking about their diets, they initially focused on what to eat on match morning. Later this was expanded to what to eat on the night before. If you have paid the proper attention to recovery, then preparation for the match is, for the most part, already taken care of. Building up muscle glycogen stores for the game happens as soon as the last training session finishes, starting Thursday night rather than Friday night in most cases. In Chapter 4.1 you will see that a further 24–36 hours of rest on a high-carbohydrate intake will top up your muscle fuel stores to see you through the game.

One note of caution—make sure that you can identify real carbohydrate sources both in everyday and pre-match settings. The foods that many footballers choose on Friday nights—chocolate, fish and chips, and oily lasagne, to name a few—are often higher in fat than carbohydrate.

### The pre-game meal

The pre-game meal has been a great point of tradition and superstition over the years, with the old guard proposing that steak and eggs were a 'real man's' meal. Although a high-fat meal like this may not seem an obvious disadvantage to all players, today's science advocates that a low-fat high-carbohydrate meal be on the pre-game menu. Read Chapter 4.3 for suggestions. If you have an afternoon or evening game you may be able to eat a bigger meal earlier in the day and finish with a ligher snack two hours before the match. Experiment to find the meal arrangement that suits you.

### Fluid intake during training and matches

With the lengthening of seasons, training sessions and pre-season matches are now conducted in warm to hot weather. But even in winter, players should be on guard against dehydration. Football tradition has seen fluid and electrolyte practices that are now known to be quite wrong—and even dangerous. Hopefully there are few football clubs in these enlightened times that promote salt tablets to prevent cramp, or think that training without fluid intake 'toughens up' players. Water bottles should always be on hand during training sessions and matches. The breaks between quarters provide more opportunities to take in fluid during the game. Read Chapter 4.4 to remind yourself of good fluid intake practices.

Extra benefits to performance may accrue from using a carbohydrate-based drink during a match. For running players this may supplement depleted muscle glycogen stores towards the end of the match, and keep blood glucose levels steady for optimum central nervous system function. Cordial or a sports drink is commonly provided by many football clubs between quarters, and in sufficient quantities these can meet both fluid and carbohydrate opportunities. We look forward to studies of carbohydrate intake during a real-life game to see if a performance boost can be detected.


PROFILE
*Drinking to your sports success*

Alcohol intake was studied among players from a top club in the Australian Football League. The information was collected in a number of ways to provide support for the results. Fifty-four players took part in a large dietary study which required them to keep an accurate food record over a typical seven-day period during the season. This record included all alcohol consumed during this time, and players were instructed to eat (and drink) as normal. The players were then interviewed in person and questioned about their usual drinking patterns. Finally, since people often under-report or over-exaggerate their alcohol intake on questionnaires, an independent assessment was devised. Blood alcohol was measured in blood samples taken from 41 players at a Sunday morning training session between 9–10am. The readings were used to gauge the alcohol consumed on the previous evening, after the match.

The football club policy encouraged that no alcohol be drunk during the week. Most players reported that they abided by this rule and drank on weekends only, on Saturday nights after the game and Sundays. However, they made up for the week's abstinence on these occasions, claiming that heavy alcohol intake was part of team bonding and unwinding after the game. During the off-season, without the club policy in effect, the frequency of alcohol binges would increase. Only five of the footballers interviewed described themselves as non-drinkers.

From the food records it was calculated that an average of 20g of alcohol was consumed by each player per day, amounting to 3.5 per cent of their total energy intake. While this sounds moderate on paper, the 'average' figure covers up for the heavy drinking on weekends. Players who consumed alcohol on the Saturday night, drank an average of 120g or twelve standard drinks (see Figure 1.6). Individual intakes ranged from 37g of alcohol to 368g—almost 40 standard drinks. In an extreme case alcohol provided 43 per cent of the kilojoules consumed that day, but on average supplied almost one-fifth of total energy intake on the Saturday.

The results of the blood alcohol readings support the Saturday night binge story. Fourteen players were recorded with positive blood alcohol readings at 10am the next morning, ranging from 0.001 to 0.113g/ml. Four players had blood alcohol readings that were over '.05' (0.05g/ml)—the legal limit for driving a car in the State of Victoria. Clearly, a lot of alcohol had been consumed by some players over the previous evening.

You might ask how professional athletes, paid to perform at their best, could have such an unprofessional attitude to alcohol misuse. The major problems are football tradition and peer group influence that support these practices. And the major obstacle to change is the 'everybody does it' excuse—a poor rationalisation at best.

Other illogical rationalisations include: 'I only do it once a week'; 'it's part of cultivating team spirit'; 'beer is good for carbos'; and 'I can sweat it out the next day'. Read Chapter 1.6 for the facts about alcohol and sports performance. In football, the most serious outcomes of binge drinking are:

Short-term:   dehydrates players who are possibly already dehydrated; exacerbates soft tissue and bruising injuries, a big part of a contact sport

Long-term:   adds to weight problems, not only by adding its own kilojoules, but by causing players to relax their attitude to other nutritional matters over the weekend.

If you spend enough time around a football club you will hear the stories about players who have missed important matches because of the lethal combination of a 'corked thigh' and a 'few' celebratory drinks after the previous match, and the players who return form the end-of-season trip seven kilograms over their playing weight.

Just because it is difficult to shift ground doesn't mean that individual players and football clubs can't push towards a more sensible approach to alcohol use. For a start:

• change the club policy on alcohol to remove the 'all or none' principle. It would be better for players to learn to drink a glass or two daily, rather than save it up for a weekend binge. Demystify the practice!

• make sure that all club functions and activities provide low alcohol and non-alcoholic drinks.

• create good role-models. Emphasise good players who have a moderate and healthy approach to alcohol intake—it is not necessary to give up alcohol altogether.

The results will be worth the effort!


## PROFILE: RODNEY
*Losing kilos and gaining metres*

At 29 years, Rodney was one of the oldest players at his top league club. He had enjoyed a successful career and been part of a number of premierships. However, in the past year Rodney had become slow, even for a backline player. At least some of this was due to a gain of body fat, a stubborn increase of four or five kilograms over his best playing weight. In the middle of pre-season, the club fitness advisor brought some scales and skinfold calipers to training. Rod clocked in at 90kg and a total skinfold sum of 93mm (not a good position to be in when your contract has yet to be renewed!).

Rod consulted the club dietitian who instructed him to keep an accurate record of all food and drinks consumed during the next seven-day period. His average daily intake of energy and nutrients was estimated (see the 'Before' column in the following table).

The dietitian focused on fat and alcohol as expendable energy sources for achieving weight loss. She explained the importance of carbohydrate foods in promoting recovery between training sessions and advised Rod to actually increase his present carbohydrate intake. Rod admitted that the hard training sessions already left him tired, and was pleased that he could lose body fat without adding to this fatigue.

A meal plan was organised to cut back fat and oil intake. Rod's wife was enthusiastic to include all the family in this plan. Ideas included:

- switching to a lower-fat milk
- cooking with a minimum of fat or oil
- using a lighter spread of margarine on toast and bread
- choosing the leanest cuts of meat and chicken, and removing all fat and skin
- cutting the protein serve at dinner to two-thirds the old size, and having one slice of meat or cheese in each sandwich at lunch instead of thick layers of both
- when having take-aways at the weekend, choosing lower-fat types and having a small serve only.

Extra carbohydrate foods were added, including a generous serve of rice, pasta or potatoes at the evening meal. Snacks now came in the form of fresh fruit or from cakes and slices made with low-fat recipes. Rod made a great effort with his alcohol intake, limiting his drinking to a couple of cans of beer at the weekends. He often managed to make this a lower alcohol beer as well.

The results were immediate. Within six weeks, Rod had lost the five kilograms he desired. As proof of his long-term commitment to this healthy eating plan, another food record was kept six months later. His new diet showed a complete change in energy and nutrient intake (see the 'After' column in the table). Rod's body weight was re-

**Rod's healthy weight loss diet—average daily intake**

|  |  | Before | After |
|---|---|---|---|
| Energy | kilojoules | 15 500 | 13 000 |
|  | Calories | 3 705 | 3 115 |
| Protein | grams | 117 | 116 |
|  | % of energy | 12.5% | 15% |
| Fat | grams | 154 | 91 |
|  | % of energy | 40 % | 27% |
| Carbohydrate | grams | 291 | 430 |
|  | % of energy | 31.5% | 56% |
| Alcohol | grams | 86 | 11 |
|  | % of energy | 16% | 2% |
| Vitamins and minerals |  | All above RDI levels | All above RDI levels and greater than before |

**Comparison of footballers' (low carbohydrate) diet and triathletes' (high carbohydrate) food selections**

| Food group | Footballers (serves/day) | Triathletes (serves/day) |
|---|---|---|
| Bread and cereals | Equivalent to 8.5 slices of bread (mostly white) | Equivalent to 18 slices of bread (mostly wholemeal) |
| Meats and protein foods | Equivalent to 300g | Equivalent to 150g |
| Dairy products | Equivalent to 600ml of milk (mostly high-fat types) | Equivalent to 800ml of milk (mostly low-fat types) |
| Added fats and oils | Equivalent to 65g | Equivalent to 20g |
| Fruit and starchy vegetables | Equivalent to 5 pieces | Equivalent to 12 pieces |

measured at 85kg and his skinfold sum at 59mm. He reported feeling full of energy and with an extra 'metre' of pace in the games. His family are now pleased to spend Sundays together, without him nursing a headache from the night before. As for the club, they are expecting a few good years out of him yet!

*Carbohydrate all week round*

Ideally, footballers should face the daily challenge of recovery from each match or training session by eating a high-carbohydrate diet all week round. Does this happen in real life? The dietary survey of the top league football club mentioned before, says no. Fifty-four players kept accurate food records for a typical seven-day period during the season. The average energy and nutrient intake of a footballer was estimated from these records with the average daily energy intake being 14 200 kilojoules (3395 Cals).

Carbohydrate provided an average of 44 per cent of total energy intake with fat providing another 37 per cent These proportions are identical to the typical Australian diet. Not only is fat intake higher than nutrition experts recommend for good health, but it is providing energy intake at the expense of carbohydrate foods, and depriving the footballer of the opportunity to replenish fuel stores each day.

A similar study conducted on a group of elite triathletes found that these athletes chose their foods quite differently to provide 60 per cent of their total energy intake from carbohydrate foods. A quick summary of the two groups shows the differences in food patterns— see the following table. While both groups ate foods from each of the major food categories, the success of the triathletes was due to:

- emphasising the serve size of the carbohydrate food rather than the protein food
- choosing the low-fat versions of foods, and preparing meals with the minimum of added fats and oils.

Footballers could learn from these patterns!

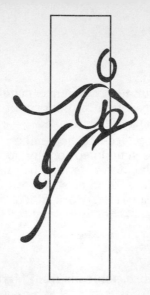

# Rugby League

Rugby League is the most popular football code in New South Wales and Queensland, with Australia's largest competition, the New South Wales Rugby League being composed of teams from these two states as well as Canberra. Competition starts at the school level, with modified rules in place to prevent injuries during scrums.

A Rugby League team consists of 13 players, six forming the forward pack and the rest making up the backline. In most leagues two reserves are allowed, but once a substitution takes place no further replacements can be made. The game, dominated by short bursts of running and heavy tackling, is basically a game of strength, skill and speed. A game takes place over two halves lasting forty minutes each.

### Training

Like Australian Rules Football, the Rugby League year is broken into three phases: pre-season, competition and off-season. Again, the length of these phases will depend on the competition level, with the top professional teams following this typical pattern:

- Off-season: may be as short as a month. There is usually a break from all team training during this time, although some players may do their own conditioning work. At lower levels, a prolonged off-season can be a time of loss of fitness and gain of body fat.
- Pre-season: can start in late November-early December. Includes running and weights, often specifically set for each player or each

227

playing position. Four to six practice matches may be played in January and February, often in the form of a pre-season competition prior to the main league.

- Competition season: March to September. Typically four to five training sessions are scheduled for the six days between games. Some sessions are devoted to strength training, while others will involve running, drills and other skill work. Training is held in the late afternoon, typically after work, since most players also work in full-time employment. Sessions may last from 1–2¹/₂ hours.

### Competition

The NSW Rugby League season runs from March to August with the final series being held in September. Each team plays one game each weekend, with Saturday and Sunday afternoons being the traditional game time. Some games are played on Monday and Friday nights. With the supplementary pre-season competition, and the 'State of Origin' series that runs in mid-season, some players compete in almost 30 matches each year.

Periodically, an international tour may be organised, sending an Australian representative side to play games against English and French teams. This poses a great challenge to the elite players involved, requiring them to extend their competition peak right through two domestic seasons.

Rugby League, being a game of short bursts of play, is not demanding in terms of energy considerations. Fuel stores are not expected to be depleted during a game, provided that muscle glycogen levels have been successfully restored since the previous game, and maintained over the week of training. However, the game is physically challenging due to injuries, soft tissue damage and bruising, caused by heavy body contact and tackling.

### Physical characteristics

Rugby League forwards are built to run the ball offensively and to tackle. The typical forward is heavy—with large muscle mass and a higher body-fat level than his backline counterpart. Backs are typically 10–20kg lighter, and in keeping with the running requirements of their game, have lower body-fat levels.

It is interesting to compare the typical physical characteristics of players in different football codes. In general, the average Rugby League player is heavier but shorter than an Australian Rules Football player, and both heavier and taller than a soccer player—reflecting the importance of muscle bulk and strength in the game of Rugby. Body-fat levels of the Rugby League player are generally higher than that of soccer players and Australian Rules Footballers, since greater aerobic fitness and mobility is required in the latter football codes.

## Other comments

Many of the comments made about Australian Rules Football apply equally to Rugby League. Until recently, tradition has played a stronger part in determining training and competition practices than have sports science principles. Peer influence and mateship have also played a strong role in this code. Hopefully, the continued development of professionalism and science-based coaching amongst Rugby teams will increase the interest in better eating—and drinking—practices amongst players.

## Common nutrition issues

Rugby League and Australian Rules Football share many nutrition concerns. Read the Australian Rules Football chapter, and the common nutrition issues (1–9) that are presented there. Special attention should be paid to the discussions concerning alcohol intake, and general nutrition knowledge and cooking skills.

In general, single players living outside a family situation are at high risk of poor nutrition. Lack of nutrition knowledge and cooking skills can be compounded by lack of time and post-training fatigue, making irregular meals and fast foods an easy pattern to fall into. As in the case of Tim below, dietary counselling can help players to find their way around the supermarket and kitchen. An astute football club will screen its team to identify players in need of nutrition education and support. Why waste talent simply because of poor eating habits?

Nutritional tradition or folklore in Rugby League is similar to Australian Rules Football, with many players still believing in high protein intakes during the week and some players continuing with pre-match meals of steak and eggs. Even more enlightened players still think of carbohydrate as a pre-game or night-before concern. Read the Australian Rules chapter, and for more detailed information about the optimum training diet, refer to Chapters 1 and 2 in Part I.

Although the fuel requirements of a Rugby League game are less than that of Australian Rules Football, optimum carbohydrate intake for training and competing in Rugby league may not be provided in a typical Australian diet—both in terms of amount and timing of intake. As in Australian Rules Football, eating carbohydrate immediately following a game or heavy training session can help to promote recovery. When muscle damage has occurred—a feature to be expected in such a heavy body contact sport—even higher carbohydrate intake is required to help refill muscle fuel stores. Carbohydrate eaten soon after the finish of exercise is better stored as muscle glycogen than carbohydrate in later meals (see Chapter 5.2).

Another issue of importance in Rugby League as well as Australian Rules Football is:

### Fluid intake during the game and training

The extended Rugby season means that training sessions and matches may be held in hot weather. With large muscle mass, and perhaps a relatively high body-fat level, Rugby League players might be expected to have poorer heat tolerance than other athletes. Heavy jumpers and/or padding can also trap heat and add to heat stress problems.

While some players still need to improve their drinking practices during the game, training often presents the greater threat for dehydration and heat stress. In summer particularly, teams may conduct prolonged and intense training sessions in the hot afternoon sun, with little regard for sweat losses. Even in winter, fluid losses should be taken into account: the tradition of toughening players by withholding fluids during training is both unscientific and unsafe. Changing to good fluid intake habits may require the updating of attitudes of players and coaching staff, as well as practical arrangements at training to make drinks available during and after training as well as games.

Water is a suitable drink in most situations. The match requirements of Rugby League do not necessitate carbohydrate intake during the game. However, if available, cordial or a sports drink can also satisfactorily supply fluid needs during a match and should not disadvantage players. After an exhausting game or training session, these carbohydrate drinks will come into their own by providing both for fluid and fuel recovery needs.

Issues that warrant additional comment for Rugby League are as follows:

### Bulking-up

Muscle mass and strength play a greater role in Rugby League than in Australian Rules Football and soccer, and bulking-up may be a priority of training and eating goals. Some teams assign a playing weight for their players and considerable effort may be required during pre-season to live up to this expectation. Read Chapters 3.6 and 3.7 for hints on bulking-up. You will need to be committed to a high energy intake from nutritious foods. This might sound great, but it is often hard work to fit frequent meals and snacks into a busy lifestyle of work and training.

### Nutrition during injury

At some stage in their sports career, most athletes suffer an injury that restricts or stops their training or competition for some time.

Injuries are double-sided in body contact sports such as Rugby League—it is not just what you do to yourself in training or a game, but what other players inflict on you as well.

Nutritional considerations during injury and rehabilitation can vary between situations and individuals. Firstly, changes in energy expenditure need to be taken into account, particularly if the lay-off off exercise is extended. An injured athlete may not automatically reduce food intake to match the sudden drop in exercise level. This can result in a significant increase in body-fat levels, making the job of rehabilitation and return to form more difficult.

Muscle mass will be lost when strength-training athletes take time off weights work, or when surgery requires body parts to be immobilised. In the latter situation, muscle atrophy can become quite pronounced. Bulking-up principles of training and eating may be needed during rehabilitation (see Chapters 3.6 and 3.7). In any case, it is important to eat nutritiously while recovering from injury. Severe injury or extensive surgery will significantly increase requirements for energy, protein and other nutrients—and inadequate nutritional support will delay recovery.

Even with the best of intentions, many injured athletes find it difficult to look after their nutritional needs. Limited mobility can interfere with normal shopping and cooking activities. Injuries to the head and neck can also directly interfere with food intake, particularly if chewing and swallowing are restricted. A fractured jaw poses a special challenge—to achieve nutritional needs while eating through a straw for six to eight weeks. Liquid meal supplements and nutritious milk drinks play a crucial role under these circumstances, and in other situations when eating or preparing solid food is difficult. See a sports dietitian for specialised help.

PROFILE: TIM
*Learning to cook in four easy steps*

Tim was in his second year at a top Rugby League team. Being recruited from a country zone meant relocating to the city, a move made easier in the first year by boarding with a family. The next year however, Tim moved into a house with a friend from work, and an ideal domestic situation it was not. Tim had been too well looked after by his Mum, and then his housemother, and his only household experience to date had been to make his bed.

After six weeks of pre-season training, it was clear that something was amiss. Tim had lost 4kg, was well under his normal playing weight, and his training performances were sluggish. The club doctor sent him to a sports dietitian to see where the problem lay.

It was only after her assessment that the full picture of Tim's eating pattern—or perhaps more correctly the lack of an eating pattern—

became apparent. The first problem to be discovered was a lack of food in the house. Tim and his housemate had not organised regular shopping expeditions. Instead, they made sporadic trips to the supermarket when motivated and midnight trips to the 7-Eleven when desperate. With no schedule of food buying, Tim would often confront the breakfast table to find no milk, no bread and Weetbix dust in the bottom of the packet.

Thus breakfast was often eaten from the vending machine in the lobby at work, or from the biscuit barrel in the tea room. In order to leave work early for training, Tim had only a half-hour break for lunch. This was well-spent in the sandwich bar next to work, but there was a limit to how much could be chewed in 30 minutes.

The next opportunity to eat was after training, and Tim admitted to often being too tired to eat, let alone cook. He estimated that it was only twice a week that he found the food and the energy to cook a real meal. His cooking repertoire was, in his own words, 'nothing flash'—sausages, steak or chops, with mashed potatoes and peas. On other nights he made toasted sandwiches or opened a tin of soup. From the financial viewpoint he tried to limit take-aways to weekends, and kept the dial-a-pizza number beside the telephone for these occasions.

'Pretty disorganised' was Tim's own comment, followed by 'How can I learn to cook?'.

The dietitian agreed that Tim's food intake was hit and miss, and that it was missing his nutritional needs in terms of total kilojoules and carbohydrate, and possibly other nutrients as well. The following plan was offered—not just to improve Tim's cooking skills but to work on his domestic organisation. Even if you are a culinary genius, it is difficult to cook a meal when your food pantry resembles that of old Mother Hubbard.

---

## STEPS TO QUICK AND HEALTHY COOKING

Step 1: shop well

- Organise regular shopping expeditions. Non-perishable items may only need to be stocked up every now and again, but plan for a weekly trip to buy perishable foods
- Shop from a list to ensure that you spend your time and money efficiently. It can be useful to keep a checklist of supplies inside the pantry door, to prompt you as you make your shopping list. The table on the following page provides some ideas, including a list of handy foods that can be stored for long periods and restocked periodically. These foods provide a great start for quick and nutritious meals.

Step 2: learn a couple of meal ideas and vary the themes

Quick and easy high-carbohydrate meals include the following themes:

*Traditional 'meat and three vegies'*

- Make these meals lower in fat by choosing lean and trimmed cuts of meat, fish or chicken. Cook with the minimum of added fats or oils.

- Break tradition by keeping to a medium serve of these protein foods, and bumping up your carbohydrate intake with a generous serve of oven- or microwave-baked potatoes, corn-on-the-cob, or side serves of rice or quick-cook noodles.

- Frozen vegies are a great time saver—no preparation, no wastage and no worries about them spoiling in the fridge before you can eat them. Not only do they come in individual varieties, but new 'mixed vegetable' combinations can add plenty of colour and nutritional variety to meals. Use fresh or frozen vegies to suit your needs.

*Versatile all-in-one-pot sauces*

- Take a base sauce—a commercial pasta sauce, or add your own herbs and spices to tinned tomatoes or tomato puree

- Add some protein—diced lean meat or chicken, tinned fish and seafood, or beans (brown the meat or chicken pieces before adding to the sauce)

- Complete by adding vegies—fresh or frozen, chopped or diced.

- Make it chunky, like a casserole and serve with rice or noodles.

- Less chunky, it can be used as a sauce for pasta or a filling for giant baked potatoes.

- Experiment with the various combinations of ingredients

*Stir-fries*

- Take the vegetable and protein combinations as above, and cut them into quick-cooking size pieces. Dry fry in a wok or large frying pan.

- Add a commercial sauce or flavour sachet for a short cut, or add your own herbs and spices as you grow confident.

- Lastly, add noodles or rice that have been cooked and drained.

*Home-made pizza*

- A high-carbohydrate pizza base can be made from bread dough and commercial pizza doughs, or for a ready-to-go pizza, use pita or Lebanese bread.

- Spread with tomato paste or commercial pasta sauces and add your own low fat toppings, such as vegies, a little lean meat, chicken or seafood.
- Spinkle cheese lightly over the top—reduced-fat mozzarellas are available.

Step 3: use healthy eating recipes to add to your repertoire

- Use healthy nutrition recipe books to expand your cooking horizons. The table on p. 236 lists some recipe books that cater for high-carbohydrate, low-fat meals—some are even specifically written for athletes.
- If you have the time and the right ingredients, you may wish to follow a recipe right through. Alternatively, just by reading through recipe books you may pick up ideas to jazz up your own cooking —particularly to learn about herbs, spices and other flavourings.

Step 4: put time-saving tricks into practice

- In a group household it makes sense to share the cooking and shopping duties amongst similarly motivated housemates.
- If you are living alone or looking after your own meals, it pays to take some cooking short-cuts—particularly for nights when you arrive home late and tired.
  - use the less busy times of the week to catch up on cooking— e.g. nights off training or quiet times on weekends. It may be possible to prepare the week's meals at one go—refrigerating or freezing the food until you need it.
  - Many recipes—especially casseroles, soups and sauces—lend themselves to leftovers. It can be just as quick to cook up a double batch. What you don't eat on one night can be reheated the following night(s), or frozen into 'single serve' portions for a rainy day.

# CHECKLIST FOR A WELL-STOCKED PANTRY AND FRIDGE

Handy foods for long-life storage
  Skim milk powder
  Wholegrain breakfast cereals
  Rolled oats
  Canned beans—baked beans, bean mix, kidney beans etc.
  Packets of beans and lentils
  Two-minute noodles
  Wholemeal rice
  Pasta and noodle varieties
  Canned salmon and tuna (in water/brine)
  Canned seafood—crab meat, mixed seafood etc.
  Pasta sauces
  Canned soups—especially low salt and main meal varieties
  Canned tomatoes, tomato puree, tomato paste
  Canned corn and champignons
  Rice cakes
  Sustagen or Exceed Sports Nutrition Supplement
  Herbs and spices

Medium-term freezer storage
  Frozen vegetables—single varieties and mixed vegetable
    combinations
  Bread
  Skim and low fat milk
  Low-fat icecream
  Meat, fish, poultry

Perishable food items for short storage
  Fruit juice
  Skim and low fat milk
  Bread
  Fresh fruit
  Fresh vegies
  Meat, fish, poultry
  Eggs
  Low-fat yoghurt
  Cottage cheese
  Reduced-fat cheese
  Margarine or butter (shouldn't need to be replaced often)

RECIPE BOOKS BASED ON HIGH-CARBOHYDRATE,
LOW-FAT EATING

*The Athlete's Kitchen* Nancy Clark (Bantam Books)
*Family Food* Gabriel Gaté (Anne O'Donovan)
*Fitness Food* (Better Living collections)
*Food for Sport Cookbook* Karen Inge and Chris Roberts (Simon &
    Schuster)
*Good Food Fast* Gabriel Gaté (Anne O'Donovan)
*Guide to Healthy Eating*, National Heart Foundation, Vols 1 and 2
*The Health and Energy Cookbook* Rosemary Stanton (Murdoch Books)
*It's only Natural* Suzanne Porter (Viking O'Neil)
*Simply Healthy* Suzanne Porter (Greenhouse)
*Smart Food* Gabriel Gaté (Anne O'Donovan)
*Taste of Life* Julie Stafford (Greenhouse and Viking O'Neil)

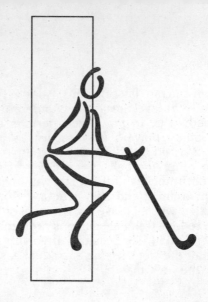

# Soccer and field hockey

Soccer and field hockey are team games played on rectangular fields—
the soccer field being slightly larger than a hockey field—with the
usual playing surface being grass or artificial turf. They share a
common link in having eleven players on a team (ten mobile players
and a goal-keeper) and in being high-intensity intermittent exercise.
Games are played in two halves of 45 minutes (soccer) and 35 minutes (hockey) with a short break between halves.

While there are both male and female competitions in each sport,
the male competition dominates in soccer with both Olympic and
World Cup status. Hockey is represented by both male and female
competitions at the Olympic Games and conducts World Champion-
ships/Cups for both sexes.

## Training

With games played in seasons, training will vary between the off-
season, pre-season and competition itself. The Australian soccer scene
now sees year-round play, with the National League being conducted
over the summer months and State/club competitions continuing as
winter sports. Hockey is predominantly played as a winter sport.

At low levels of competition in both sports, players may have

237

extensive off-season lay-offs and relatively short pre-season preparation. Body-fat levels may be considerably higher at the beginning of each season, due to prolonged periods of inactivity. Even at the elite level, many players may return to pre-season training with significant losses in both fitness and body condition.

As in the other football codes covered in this book, pre-season training in both hockey and soccer will involve general conditioning work, weight training and skill practice. Concentration on skills and match practice will increase as the season approaches. During the season, two to four training sessions are generally scheduled between matches, with mid-week sessions involving lengthy match practice, and the end of the week seeing a gradual easing-off in training load to prepare for the next match.

### Competition

The competition season generally provides a weekly match, with the national competition in soccer also involving team travel, and some mid-week and double-header fixtures. Soccer and hockey may also be played in tournaments of one to several weeks, with a heavy schedule of matches. At the international level, extensive travel may also be involved in competition tours.

Hockey and soccer are played as fast games of intensive play, with light activity between bursts. While rules restrict the amount of tackling and body contact that is permitted, both games can have a significant component of physical contact, with the potential for contact injuries. Time-motion studies of soccer have determined that the average distance covered per match by national and international level players is about ten kilometres. This of course will vary between positions on the field, as well as the level of competition. However, studies have also reported that the main difference between players of different levels is not in the total distance covered, but in the speed of play, the length of maximal bursts and the number of tackles and headings. Goalkeepers have been estimated to cover about four kilometres in the course of a match, with this activity level partly accounted for by the necessity to maintain arousal.

Games that are played under hot conditions, as well as drawing heavily on fuel stores, will challenge the fluid stores of players. While 1–2kg fluid losses have been reported during standard soccer games, under hot humid conditions sweat losses have been reported at double this level.

### Physical characteristics

Hockey and soccer players, as well as being skilled, must be agile and fast. Players vary widely in body size, and differences in physical characteristics may not so much limit performance, as determine position on the field or style of play. While most players tend to be well-muscled, regardless of height and weight characteristics, a low body-fat level is also an advantage for speed and agility.

**Typical physique (elite hockey players)**

|  | Male | Female |
|---|---|---|
| Height | 175–186cm | 161–171cm |
| Weight | 71–80kg | 55–69kg |
| Skinfold sum | 40–60mm | 59–83mm |

**Typical physique (elite soccer players)**

|  | Male |
|---|---|
| Height | 176–187cm |
| Weight | 72–87kg |
| Skinfold sum | 43–58mm |

## Common nutrition issues

### Body-fat levels

So you have the skill to be a good hockey or soccer player, but you're lacking a little in speed and stamina. Could it be that you are carrying extra weight that you don't need? Perhaps after a good rest over the off-season you have returned almost twice the player you used to be. Or perhaps, as in the case of Michael below, an injury has kept you inactive and in energy imbalance. At some time in your playing career you may find yourself battling the bulge.

For healthy and permanent fat-loss methods, read Chapter 3. And for year-round weight control, be aware of changes in your energy requirements. At the end of the season, you may need to significantly reduce your food intake to match the decrease in training output—or alternatively you may choose to keep up some activity to give you a head-start on next season.

### The training diet—week-round recovery

Recovery between matches is difficult when a heavy training load is carried out on the intervening days. A soccer study has reported that muscle glycogen levels of players recovered very slowly in the days after the match, due to a combination of inadequate carbohydrate intake and continued training. Damage to muscle fibres arising from the match may also slow down the rate of glycogen storage.

The traditional approach of 'carbohydrates at the end of the week' is no longer appropriate for hockey and soccer players, who need a

239

daily intake of carbohydrates to continually replenish their muscle stores. Read Chapters 1 and 2 for an overview of all aspects of the training diet, but pay special attention to the idea of a high- carbohydrate intake every day. This will keep you in constant recovery mode—avoiding mid-week slumps and progressive fatigue over the season.

### Match preparation

With a good recovery diet in week-round practice, muscle fuel stores should gradually increase over the week. Light training at the end of the week, and the continuation of high-carbohydrate meals, will top-up muscle and liver glycogen stores as much as possible. Read Chapter 4.2 for general ideas, and make sure that your carbohydrate meals are as high in carbohydrate as you think. Chapters 1.3 and 2.2 provide practical ideas about carbohydrate foods.

The pre-match meal is eaten to top up carbohydrate stores on the day of the event and to make sure that fluid levels are looked after. You should experiment with the type, timing and amount of food that suits your game schedule and individual preferences. Don't let match nerves and travel requirements interfere with what you need, and if a certain meal suits you—regardless of how 'scientific' it seems—then stick to what you like. Most players have adopted high-carbohydrate low-fat meals but for others the tradition of the high-protein (and high-fat) meal dies hard. The most important aspect of the pre-event meal is that you feel comfortable and confident with your choice.

See Chapter 4.4 for more details, and see how Leon successfully solved his match day food later in this chapter.

### Match considerations

Soccer and hockey matches place reasonable demands on both the fluid and carbohydrate stores of its players, particularly when there is a carry-over effect from matches played in close proximity (e.g. a tournament or mid-week fixture). Soccer studies have reported low muscle glycogen levels in players after a match—sometimes with significant depletion occurring by half time. Low muscle glycogen levels are likely to interfere with both endurance and high intensity exercise capacity—and indeed in these studies, players with depleted muscle glycogen stores had a slower average speed and covered less ground than their team-mates in the second half of the match.

Measurements on first-class soccer players have also shown that at least some players finish the game with low blood-sugar levels. It has been speculated that such a condition could impair the speed and accuracy of mental processing—and thus skill level.

In accordance with these results, some soccer studies have reported an improvement in match performance when carbohydrate is consumed just prior to the game as well as during half-time. The effect has been attributed to both an improvement in movement during the second half of the game (better muscle carbohydrate availability) as well as better skills/less mistakes during this period (prevention of central nervous system fatigue).

With sweat losses during the match requiring fluid replacement strategies—particularly for matches played in hot conditions—carbohydrate drinks could be of value as a match drink. Drinking between 500–1000ml of sports drink or cordial, at a carbohydrate concentration of about 5–7 per cent, will provide for both fluid and carbohydrate needs simultaneously (see Chapter 4.7). Experiment in training and practice matches to see whether this appears to be of benefit. The carbohydrate may be unnecessary for your particular game, but is unlikely to interfere with fluid balance if it has passed the training test. Nevertheless you may decide to stick to plain water if the carbohydrate seems unwarranted.

In very hot conditions, such as the tropics, it may be necessary to replace considerably more fluid than half-time drinks will allow. It may be possible to have extra drink bottles at the side of the field for a quick sip between plays. Take extra care to drink before and after matches so that you start the game well-hydrated.

*Post-match recovery*

Recovery should begin straight after the match—a time that is most often swallowed up in celebrations, commiserations or general relaxation, rather than careful attention to nutritional needs. But with the next match a maximum of six days away, and a training session scheduled in 24–48 hours, carbohydrate and fluid losses need immediate attention (see Chapter 5 for an explanation of the role of timing in recovery after exhaustive exercise).

Organise to have suitable drinks and snacks available after the match as a team activity so that everyone can enjoy the benefits. A post-match spread of sandwiches, fruit, soup and carbohydrate drinks in the club, or a box of supplies in the bus on the way back from 'away' matches can get recovery off to a good start. Players can make their own decisions about the rest of the evening's activities—whether it be discos or take-aways—hopefully taking heed of the club lesson on priorities.

*Alcohol intake*

There is a tendency in team sports to celebrate matches with alcohol intake—and unfortunately more alcohol intake than is good for sports performance. Read Chapter 1.6 to learn about the sensible use of alcohol in sport, particularly in post-match recovery. There is no need to be a teetotaller, but neither can excessive intake (even once a week with 'everyone' doing it) be condoned as professional behaviour. Take special care with bruising and soft tissue injuries that occur in a match or match practice. A good dose of alcohol will significantly increase the damage and prolong the time for recovery and rehabilitation.

### Tournaments and travelling

Hockey and soccer tournaments may involve many games in quick succession, placing great importance on the recovery strategies already discussed. The plan, in a nutshell, is to recover as quickly after a match as possible, to continue to rebuild muscle glycogen stores between matches, and to supply additional fluid and carbohydrates during matches. Each of these strategies will take on greater importance as the tournament continues.

Of course, when the competition means being away from home or travelling on a tour, the challenge becomes greater and being organised becomes imperative. For help as a travelling athlete, read the account in the Tennis chapter.

PROFILE: MICHAEL
*Injury—frustration and fat gain*

Michael couldn't believe that in three months his hockey career had turned from bright to uncertain, and his body from trim and taut to, well, cuddly. The irony was that he had spent most of his teen years as a bean pole, able to put anything into his mouth and never gain a gram. It was only in recent years of heavy training and weight work that his body had filled out. Then, in the past ten weeks while nursing a tibial stress fracture, his skinfolds had climbed from 47mm to 81mm, and his weight had rocketed by 7kg.

At his latest medical check, the doctor had ordered him to see the clinic dietitian, warning that the extra weight was not only bad for his game but that it put extra load on his weakened leg. It was likely that this had already delayed his recovery. After the usual six-week rest he had attempted to resume light training, only to suffer a recurrence of tibial pain.

Michael explained his plight to the dietitian, complaining that he had never had to worry about his weight or food intake before. Why was there suddenly a problem?

After a full assessment of the situation, the dietitian offered a simple explanation—'energy in' was greater than 'energy out: and a number of factors were operating to cause this:

- A change in metabolic rate with age. As an adolescent, Michael had burnt up many thousands of kilojoules each day to cope with the needs of growth and training. Now that this had slowed down, he needed to be a bit more careful of the 'bottomless pit' eating habits that he had learned.

- Drastic change of activity level. Playing both state and club level hockey had kept Michael busy with training or matches every day of the week. A sudden standstill in his exercise program was a major change to his lifestyle and to energy requirements. Michael admitted that he had taken things a little too easy in his rehabilitation. Although the physiotherapist had suggested swimming and cycling as alternative exercise modes, Michael had not enjoyed either and had let the program slide.

- Poor general dietary habits. Michael had always thought that if your weight was OK, then you must be eating well—and never having had to worry about his skinfold levels before, he had kept himself insulated from any advice about good nutrition practices. The dietitian assessed Michael's diet to be high in fat—deadly for kilojoule intake.

- Boredom eating and drinking. Being injured leaves a lot of time to sit around the house, feeling sorry for yourself and becoming bored. Not used to being home straight after work—usually he went to training—Michael had begun new habits of afternoon snacks and a beer after work. In fact, thinking about it, there had been quite a few commiseration sessions spent with friends at the pub. The alcohol and 'comfort foods' were sneaking in far more kilojoules than he had realised.

Michael committed himself to a full plan of rehabilitation—both for his leg and for his abdominal skinfolds. It was time to take stock of his new energy requirements, and to change his energy balance in favour of body-fat loss—at least until he could resume full training. A proper plan of swimming, upper-body weight work and cycling was organised. Not only did this burn up some kilojoules, but it kept him out of the house (and the fridge) and gave him a focus of encouragement and goal-setting. A dietary plan was written, limiting food quantities in general, and fat and oil intake in particular. A weekly quota of light beer was negotiated, although Michael suggested that he was happy to go 'on the wagon' for the rest of the season, or at least until his body fat was below 50mm again.

Within six weeks, the bulk of the body fat had been lost and Michael was back in half-training. Food quantities were adjusted as energy requirements and body-fat goals changed. The dietitian promised Michael that his food patterns were not only good for weight control, now and in the future, but with his new concentration on carbohydrate intake, he could expect action-packed training and matches. Michael can't wait to put it to the test in his first game back in two to three weeks time.

PROFILE: LEON
*The pre-event meal*

When Leon moved up into the senior team at his soccer club, his father gave him some advice: 'You'll need a lot of stamina at this level son, especially with the game kicking off at 3.00pm. When I used to play I always had a big breakfast for energy—steak, eggs and toast. I'll get your mother onto it.'

The next Sunday, Leon sat down to his father's tried and true pre-match meal. At one o'clock when they left for the ground his stomach was full of food and butterflies. In the first half he felt sick, at half-time he was sick, and in the second half he wandered around the field feeling empty and a bit tired.

The following week Leon went back to the breakfast he had eaten in his junior league days—a couple of pieces of toast and honey and some fruit juice. This was light and compact and had served him well in an 11.00am match. However eaten at 9.00am in the morning it didn't seem substantial enough to get him though an afternoon match. By midday he was feeling hungry again and by match-time it was hard to concentrate on his game above the rumbling of his stomach.

He asked the coach for some advice, and found that a sports dietitian had been organised to come to the club to talk about this very topic. With a revamped and expanded league this season, the coach was worried about having to face some new match-day conditions. The inclusion of some new clubs would mean a four-hour bus trip to some of the 'away' matches. He wondered whether he should organise a team breakfast along the road to break up the trip, or whether they should take some food supplies on the bus. Later in the year, the team might play in a country league tournament with matches at various times of the day over a week or so of competition. Should his players eat differently for morning matches to evening matches? Time for some expert advice!

The dietitian explained that the role of the pre-match meal was to tie up the loose ends of the weekly eating efforts—not to be a magic wand for performance. She asked the players to nominate whether they were happy with their present pre-match meal routines, or whether they thought there was room for improvement. About a third of the team admitted they had experienced problems at some time. Some, like Leon, had difficulties with knowing how much and at what time to eat. Others suffered with pre-game nerves to the extent that they were unable to eat anything.

The dietitian compiled a list of the types of foods chosen by the players for their pre-event meal, and presented it for discussion. There was a wide range of meal patterns, ranging from two small meals to a late-morning brunch, and from cooked breakfasts to a piece of toast. The first thing that was obvious to the players, was that each person had an individual approach to his needs—and that different plans suited different players.

The goals of the pre-event meal were outlined:

- to top-up liver and perhaps muscle glycogen stores;
- to top-up fluid levels;
- to feel comfortable (neither too full nor too hungry), and to avoid foods that disagree; and
- to feel confident and ready for action.

The most obvious way to fulfil these goals was with a high-carbohydrate meal, and the dietitian listed some suitable food combinations—from typical breakfast fare such as cereal, toast and fruit to more elaborate meals such as rice pudding, pancakes and syrup and pasta with tomato sauces. She also discussed low-carbohydrate or high-fat foods that athletes often ate as pre-event meals—including steak, bacon and eggs, and oily lasagnes.

Were these foods bad, the dietitian was asked? She agreed they fitted the tradition rather than the scientific theory of an ideal pre-game meal, but suggested that for some players they didn't seem to cause ill-effects. She recounted the tale of an American swimmer who had eaten an amazing spread of hamburgers and cookies before swimming to a gold medal, and concluded that many of the effects of the last meal were psychological as well as nutritional. It was obviously important to believe in what you had done.

Most players were interested in experimenting with the low-fat high-carbohydrate menu plans, although a couple of die-hards decided to stick to their 'lucky steaks' (eaten no doubt with their 'lucky' knives and forks). The dietitian advised that the amount and timing of meals on match morning was an individual preference also, and suggested that each player began by working from his everyday breakfast routine to find a pre-match plan. For example, someone who usually ate a hearty breakfast of cereal and six rounds of toast might need a bigger meal than someone who was satisfied with a muffin and fruit juice.

Whatever time the match was played, at least two hours pre-event was the eating schedule to work back from. For afternoon matches, the choice between a single (larger) meal and an early breakfast followed by a later snack would rest on individual comfort as well as the match travel arrangements. For home games it may not be necessary to leave for the ground until the early afternoon, whereas many of the 'away' games may mean an early departure from home. The dietitian suggested that for long trips to matches, an organised meal-stop en route could be good for team morale as well as nutrition. She suggested that a regular venue be chosen and supplied with a menu, and that a buffet format would enable players to better cater for their individual likes and needs.

What about players who needed a small top-up to breakfast, either at the ground or at home? Light snacks could include sandwiches, fruit, or a liquid meal supplement such as Sustagen or Exceed Sports Nutrition Supplement, with the liquid meals being handy for those unable to keep down any solid food. The final item to remember was fluid intake, including special attention on hot and humid days. With all players trained to drink during their stretching and warm-up to the match, hydration needs seemed to be well-looked after.

The players at Leon's club now eat their own 'secret weapon' breakfasts, and occasionally tease each other about their special pancakes or their Sustagen rituals. Nevertheless, they all know that once they take to the field they are ready for anything, with the pre-event meal being the icing on the cake of a good week's training and nutrition.

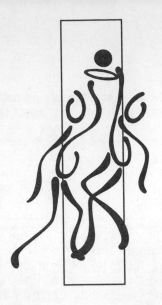

# Basketball and netball

Basketball and netball are team ball games, played both on indoor and outdoor courts. While basketball is played at a high level by both males and females, netball is predominantly a female participation sport. Strong international competition exists for both sports, with basketball being an Olympic sport.

Basketball is played by teams of up to ten players, with five players appearing on the court at one time. Each player has a specific role to play on the court, but all players are mobile—covering the whole court and being involved in both offensive and defensive plays. Players are continually substituted from the bench throughout the game. A basketball game can be played in four 12-minute quarters, or in two 20-minute halves, with a break of 10–15 minutes at half-time. Since the timing clock stops when the ball is out of play, the actual time elapsed for each game is considerably more.

A netball team is composed of seven players, each in a specific position with a defined role and a defined court space. Reserve players are allowed, but once a substitution is made a benched player cannot return to the court unless replacing an injured team-mate. A netball game can be played as a game of 15-minute quarters or two 20-minute halves, again with a short break at the half-way point.

At the elite level, both netball and basketball are fast-paced and skilled, and are both physical games, in spite of rules against direct contact between components. Considerable demands are placed upon anaerobic energy systems, with aerobic fitness assisting recovery between bursts of play.

### Training

Basketball and netball are generally played in competition seasons with national leagues existing in both sports. The competition season for the National Basketball League spreads from March to September, with the play-offs for the finals in October. Training for the next season may start soon after Christmas, leaving only a short break in between seasons. Most players at this level will remain active for the whole year, indulging in personal training when the team does not hold official practice. At lower levels, players may have longer breaks between seasons, and find themselves at risk for weight gain and loss of fitness during this time.

Elite players train on a daily basis, and in some cases—for example, training camps for national teams—twice daily sessions may be undertaken. In pre-season, the emphasis is on building a fitness base, with training involving greater amounts of running and strength work than at other times of the year. Skills work and practice matches, where set plays are developed, are practised all year round and are the dominant mode of training.

The number of training sessions undertaken each week will vary with the number of games played. The team will normally meet for three or four sessions per week, and players may train individually or in small groups at other sessions, concentrating on weaknesses and specific tasks relevant to their roles on court.

At a non-elite level, training loads vary. Many basketball and netball players simply train individually to keep fit and to practise skills, and then play in a weekly competition with perhaps one or two team training sessions a week.

### Competition

For national league competition, it is practical to divide the program into home games, and games played on tour. Home games are usually played on a Friday or Saturday night, with a single game each weekend. Tours may involve playing two or three games (Friday night, Saturday night and Sunday afternoon), often in different cities. This presents a great challenge, both in terms of recovery between games, as well as the interruption to sleep, diet and training caused by travelling.

Even at a sub-elite and recreational level, many players enjoy playing for a number of teams, or in a number of competitions, and may find themselves with a weekly commitment of two or three matches. This may pose a similar challenge of recovery against the background of a less than ideal lifestyle.

Tournament competitions, over weekends or weeks, present an even more difficult routine. Depending on the size of the competition, teams may be organised into a draw, with the winners of each zone or pool meeting in a final series.

## Physical characteristics

Height is the most noticeable physical characteristic in these ball-games—particularly in basketball, and particularly for centres and forwards. In netball, there is greater allowance for shorter players in some positions, particularly where the ball is played close to the ground. However, netball players are generally above-average height.

Lower body-fat levels are an advantage in improving agility and speed, and with assisting movement off the ground. The body-fat levels of elite players may be relatively low, reflecting both the training load as well as the advantages of being lean, however, they do not usually drop as low as those of endurance athletes. At lower levels of play it is possible to be skilled but less trim and fit.

**Typical physique (elite basketball players)**

|  | Male | Female |
| --- | --- | --- |
| Height | 190–208cm | 170–184cm |
| Weight | 87–112kg | 62–82kg |
| Skinfold sum | 53–81mm | 58–85mm |

**Typical physique (elite netball players)**

|  | Female |
| --- | --- |
| Height | 171–180cm |
| Weight | 63–76kg |
| Skinfold sum | 73–116mm |

## Common nutrition issues

### The training diet—being organised

Energy requirements in basketball and netball can be high, but reflect the size and growth needs of some players more than energy expenditure from exercise. Training and matches while a lengthy part of the day, are generally not as energy-intensive as they might appear, due to the emphasis on skill practice, and stop-start play.

A single game of netball or basketball does not provide a great threat to the fuel capabilities of a trained athlete. However, in many situations players struggle with their recovery, due to the carry-over effects of a daily schedule of training and matches. It is not just that special nutritional needs are created, such as the need for a high daily carbohydrate intake, but rather that players can find it hard to set an organised meal plan, because of their hectic and unpredictable lifestyle. The majority of training sessions and matches are generally carried out at night—and often late into the night. For those with full-time jobs, or even those who are full-time athletes, this can mean a busy day.

How do you spread your food over the day to fit exercise needs—such as not eating too close to a game—as well as fit in with the general schedule of meal-times followed by your family or the rest of the world? Juggled meals can often mean disorganised nutrition. An evening game may finish late at night, leaving the player unmotivated to cook, unable to find somewhere to eat out, or uncomfortable about eating a big meal before going to bed. Since the player may have been reluctant or unable to eat a planned meal before the game, the whole day may become a series of grabbed snacks—often poor in nutritional quality. If this is the pattern for the week, overall nutritional status can be jeopardised. Busy players may find, between games, training and basketball meetings that they only get to eat a cooked meal once a week.

The principles of training nutrition are explained in Chapters 1 and 2. The major task of most players will be to organise a meal routine that allows all goals to be met. You may need to use nights at home to catch up with cooking for the week, thus providing quick meals for game nights. You may need to experiment with the pre-game meal plan, to split your food into a pre-event snack and a post-event top-up. Snacks can be nutritious if well-planned. You might even like to switch the focus of the day to make your lunch the main meal, and have lighter meals for the rest of the day.

### Losing body fat

The beginning of the season may see you needing to lose body fat, or perhaps you are coming back from an injury. For some female players it is a constant struggle to reach an ideal playing weight. See Chapter 3 for safe and sensible ideas, and read the account of Vicki below.

### Iron status

Low iron status may be a problem for female players and some male players. Contact and impact events—hitting other players or landing hard on the floor—may increase iron losses through increased red-blood-cell destruction. In any case, female athletes and athletes on weight-loss diets are at risk of iron deficiency due to a low iron intake. See Chapter 2.5 for a discussion of iron requirements and ways to ensure a high iron intake.

## *Match preparation—the pre-event meal*

In theory, the pre-event meal should be a light, high-carbohydrate meal eaten at least two hours before the match. Experiment to find something that suits you. Since it is likely that you will play matches at various times of the day or night, you may need to be versatile with meal ideas to suit a number of occasions. See Chapter 4.4.

## *Match and training fluids*

If you are working hard, and the stadium is hot, it is possible to lose a significant amount of fluid through sweating. Look after fluid levels by drinking before training or matches, and for hot, lengthy sessions, take a water bottle to the court. And of course, rehydrate well after you have finished—especially if you have another session or match coming up soon. Water is probably adequate, but there may be no harm in trying a sports drink. See Chapter 4.6.

## *Tournament nutrition*

Tournament schedules are often challenging, setting you to play a number of matches over a short period. Travelling may also be part of the deal. As soon as you know your likely schedule of matches, begin to plan a meal routine. You will need to take into account suitable pre-event meals (Chapter 4.4), and post-event recovery strategies (Chapter 5). If you are on the move, or playing in foreign parts, then the notes on the travelling athlete will be of help (see Tennis chapter).

## *On the road again*

Being on the road for the weekend is tough work. Not only is there disruption to your normal eating, sleeping and training schedule, but you may be required to play two or three games over three days. This will challenge your skills of recovery and organisation. See the account of the Travelling Athlete in the Tennis chapter to learn a three-pronged plan of attack:

- Know your nutrition goals, including recovery (Chapter 5), pre-event meals (Chapter 4.4), and the general principles of training nutrition (Chapters 1 and 2).
- Plan ahead. You may be able to find restaurants to eat at or make some plans with your hotel to cater for the meals that you need at the time that you need them. (Remember, your pre-event and post-event meal schedule may not fit in with their normal dining room times).
- Be assertive and make things happen the way that you want them to.

Some teams leave a lot of this to be organised by a team manager or the team captain, and eat most of their meals as a team. In other clubs, players are responsible for most of their own eating and are given a *per diem*, or daily allowance, for their food. For financial and practical reasons (where else can you eat late at night) take-aways and fast foods can make up a big part of the weekend's eating. Take-aways have a bad reputation—nutritionally speaking—that is not always deserved. Read the account below to learn about fitting them into your lifestyle and your nutrition goals.

PROFILE: VICKI
*Lose body fat, once and for all!*

In one year, Vicki had lost over 20kg—that is to say, that she had lost the same two kilograms over and over. She certainly had the desire and motivation to lose weight. Her netball coach at school had rated her as a potential state-level player, but a centre cannot afford to carry extra body-fat. At sixteen, Vicki had stopped growing up, and had started to grow 'out'. Now, in Year 12, she was four kilograms heavier than at the end of last year, and she was beginning to feel and show it on the court. Her self-initiated dieting was not going anywhere. After grapefruit breakfasts and green apple lunches she would lose 1–2kg, only to put it back on in the next week. The coach insisted that a more healthy and long-term weight control program be found.

A round-table conference was held with her parents to discuss a plan of attack. Vicki's mother was enthusiastic and decided that the whole family would watch their food intake. They bought a copy of a healthy nutrition recipe book and followed the directions. Skim milk was introduced, non-fat cooking methods became the order of the day, and take-aways were banished to a monthly treat.

But even without the skin on the chicken and the chocolate biscuits, Vicki's weight remained high. It didn't seem fair—the team trained three nights a week and played on weekends, and Vicki ran for a half hour on the other days. Her best friend didn't exercise at all, ate McDonalds twice a week, and didn't have an ounce of excess fat on her body.

Vicki and her Mum eventually took the problem to a sports dietitian and were congratulated on their progress so far. The dietitian consoled Vicki that her energy needs did seem to be lower than others, but said that comparing herself to other girls would not solve the problem. Instead, she had to look at her own situation carefully, and find ways to increase energy expenditure and/or decrease energy intake from food.

The demands of school and homework did not leave much time for extra training, although Vicki agreed that she could step up her runs to 40 or 50 minutes. This meant the major solution had to come from changes in food intake. Vicki described her usual meal patterns to the dietitian, and it appeared that the family food plan already provided the right types of food. Vicki's mother questioned this carefully, saying that in her day carbohydrate foods were considered fattening and she couldn't believe the amount of bread and potatoes that the new dietary principles encouraged.

The dietitian reinforced the nutrition messages from the healthy nutrition book, and agreed that the attitude to carbohydrate had changed. She reminded them that carbohydrate foods provided the most important fuel for exercise and therefore could not be neglected. She was puzzled, though, that Vicki's serve sizes did not seem extraordinary or unreasonably large—so where was the difficulty in losing weight? Vicki was sent home to keep a food record, and that's when the problem emerged.

Even Vicki was surprised to see the number of snacks she had eaten, but the food record had captured it in black and white. The hours spent in the evenings, cramming in homework before she went to bed, were also spent in and out of the kitchen. Weekends and afternoons free from training were worse, with frequent bowls of cereal and sandwiches. Between her study and training commitments, Vicki didn't have much time for leisure, so she used food to break the boredom. It wasn't so much the types of foods that she snacked on—they were all high carbohydrate and low-fat—but that the extra kilojoules were being consumed in the name of entertainment rather than need.

The dietitian helped Vicki to reorganise her homework schedule to include blocks of study, rewarded with some real 'time out'. A list of enjoyable activities was written to give her alternatives to eating when she became bored. In addition, she was allowed to have a weekly treat—a small portion of her favourite food.

The plan worked well. Within six weeks she had lost most of the excess weight, and the dietitian was able to show her that her skinfolds had dropped by 25mm. Because she knows how she achieved these goals, and has reorganised her eating behaviour to sustain the effort, Vicki should not have any further difficulties with this weight 'finding' her again.

PROFILE
*Take-aways—fast food doesn't need to be junk food!*

When you live life in the fast lane, it is inevitable that fast food will be part of it. For athletes, take-aways may provide a quick meal after a late training session or match, or they may be part of the travelling diet when cooking facilities are not available and restaurants are out of the budget range. Maybe after a hard week of work and training, you just want a day when you don't have to exert yourself with domestic duties.

Despite their convenience, fast foods and take-aways do not generally have a good reputation. 'Junk food' is a frequent description for these foods, although that doesn't stop people from eating (or liking) them. Most people feel a little guilty about making take-aways a big part of their diet, and some people feel guilty about eating them at all. Is the reputation warranted?

Fast foods generally go against the principles of healthy nutrition and the optimum training diet. A nutritional assessment of popular take-away foods—for example, the menus at the big hamburger chains and fried chicken outlets—finds that they are high in fat, salt, sugar and kilojoules, and low in fibre and some vitamins, particularly vitamins A and C. For an athlete, many take-aways may lack sufficient carbohydrate to meet fuel needs. From the financial point of view, take-aways are more expensive than a home prepared meal, though you may not notice this on a once-off occasion. However, they are less expensive than general restaurant eating.

Thus it is likely that indiscriminate use of take-aways may prevent the athlete from achieving nutritional goals. However, this does not have to be the case. With planning and good nutrition knowledge, it is possible to let take-aways play a useful role in your diet. Use the following strategies as an overall guide.

- Limit the number of times that you eat take-aways—make use of their convenience when you really need it.
- Be selective in making your order. It is possible to make selections or modify choices so that they are more in line with the healthy nutrition guidelines.
- Have a small portion only and make up the rest of your meal with other foods. Alternatively, eat just what you need, rather than the full menu.
- Make sure that the rest of your meals compensate for mismatched nutritional goals from your fast-food meals.
- Think wider than the well-known chains. There are some 'healthy' take-away outlets being set up, and a sandwich is the quintessential healthy fast food which you can buy almost anywhere.

As a rule of thumb, choose foods that are based on carbohydrate—either bread, rice, potato or pasta. Avoid batters and deep-fried foods, and be aware that pastry is high in fat (unless it is filo pastry). Make up fillings with vegetables and salads rather than lots of protein (and fat). The following table compares some good food choices with foods that fail to meet the dietary guidelines.

# A GUIDE TO TAKE-AWAYS

| High-carbohydrate/low-fat choices | High-fat choices |
| --- | --- |
| Roll or sandwich—no margarine. Lean meat/chicken/salmon/cottage cheese/ cheese (medium serve). Plenty of salad. | Toasted ham and cheese sandwiches dripping with margarine |
| Pizza—thick crust (especially whole-meal). Vegetarian or seafood topping. Ask for less cheese. | Pizza with the lot— especially the 'meat-lovers' special' |
| Salad hamburger—one rissole, plenty of salad and wholemeal roll if possible. Watch the mayonnaise or dressings. | The Quarter-Pounder with the lot |
| Steak sandwich—as for hamburger | Crumbed schnitzel |
| Souvlaki—another version of the hamburger or other low-fat filling (bread with meat plus salad) | Pies, pasties, sausage rolls etc. |
| Baked potato with a little cheese and coleslaw or other low-fat filling (not butter or sour cream) | Chips (and fried fish etc.) |
| Chicken roll with coleslaw and corn on the cob | Deep fried chicken or chicken nuggets |
| Fruit juice | |
| Low-fat fruit smoothies (low-fat milk, icecream or yoghurt and fruit) | Thickshake |
| Low fat frozen yoghurt or Vitari | Icecream—especially extra creamy types |

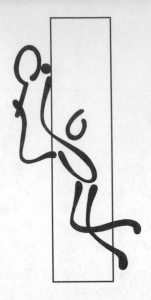

# Tennis

Tennis is played by both men and women, in singles and in doubles competition (same-sex and mixed-sex pairs), and at levels varying from a 'social hit' to the lucrative international circuit. Other variables in the game include the court surface, and whether it is located indoor or outdoors.

At an elite level, tennis is a fast and mobile game, characterised by bursts of intense exercise against a background of quiet movement. The average tennis point lasts eight seconds, with the longest points, even at the world class level, rarely lasting more than half a minute. Thus the game itself is highly reliant on anaerobic energy systems, although a developed aerobic capacity is an advantage in terms of recovery between points, stamina and tolerance to heat.

Tennis is a game of skill, speed, agility and concentration—and often, endurance. Men's matches at international tournaments are often marathon efforts of four or five hours, with long rallies for each point and many sets going to tie-breakers. While the exercise is not continuous for this duration, such a game is likely to challenge the carbohydrate fuel stores of the athlete, and require great discipline to maintain concentration.

## Training

For professional players, tennis is a full-time job. Between tournaments, 20–40 hours per week may be spent in training—with the majority of this devoted to on-court practice. Most players will supplement this with about an hour per day of off-court conditioning work, such as running, weight training and agility work. This work may vary according to different stages of preparation, and the specific weaknesses in a player's game.

Further down the competition level, tennis players will not have the luxury of hours to spend on training. Nevertheless, the balance of time available will again be spent on court practice.

## Competition

Most competitive tennis in Australia is played in the form of graded pennant competitions, with teams (four members) meeting each other in a weekly draw. A final series amongst the top finishing teams then determines the pennant winner.

The other form of tennis competition, particularly at the elite level, is tournament tennis. This begins at the sub-elite level with weekend tournaments, and continues from satellite tournaments to the elite circuit of Grand Prix and Grand Slam events. The length of the tournament varies with the number of player entries, being run as a 'cut-throat' competition where losing players are eliminated, while winners continue to the next round. The standard Grand Prix tournament, beginning with 32 or 64 entries, is held over a week, with the winner needing to win four to six matches to take out the trophy.

A tennis match is played over the best of three or five sets for men, and the best of three sets for women. The length of a match varies greatly, from 30 minutes to three hours for a three-set match, and from 80 minutes to more than five hours for a five-set competition. The fuel and fluid demands of a match will vary accordingly. However, in tournament tennis, the nutritional focus is not so much on the effects of a single match, but on the carry-over effects from playing so many matches in succession.

Tournament tennis sets an extremely tough schedule for players, requiring many to play in a single and doubles match each day—with perhaps only one rest day—until their outcome is decided. While muscle glycogen levels may survive one match, the continual daily schedule will challenge the athlete to fully recover fuel stores between matches. Depleted muscle glycogen levels will interfere with both sprint and endurance components of performance, and limit the player's ability to perform at an optimum level.

For elite tennis players, life is a continual program of tournaments and exhibition matches, with most taking only short breaks between each venture onto the circuit to recover and prepare for the next. On average, an elite player participates in twenty tournaments each year.

## Physical characteristics

Some general physical characteristics that are of value to a tennis player include long arms and a relatively low centre of gravity (short legs in proportion to the trunk). These features should assist a player, with extra reach for playing strokes and height for serving, and with greater mobility around the court.

Other physical characteristics do not so much limit performance as help determine the style of game a player can play well. For example, tall muscular players might best use their height and power with an aggressive serve and volley game, while shorter, agile players may do better with a mobile court-covering game.

In general, the body-fat levels of tennis players are relatively low, since excess body fat can reduce both stamina and heat tolerance. In women's tennis, this feature hasn't always been so. In earlier times, many top females were skilled but relatively fat and lacking in aerobic fitness. Martina Navratilova set a trend in women's tennis, by trimming her body-fat level and developing great strength and fitness, to become almost invincible during the 1980s.

### Common nutrition issues

#### Training nutrition

During the 1980s Ivan Lendl and Martina Navratilova publicised the importance of nutrition in their game preparation. Martina featured in Robert Haas' book *Eat to Win*, extolling the virtues of her new style of eating. Although some aspects of the *Eat to Win* diet run contrary to the advice in this book, the essential shared element is the encouragement to boost carbohydrate intake to fuel exercise needs, and to reduce the characteristic fat, salt and sugar intakes of the Western diet.

The testimony of these champions has influenced tennis players of all levels to consider their nutrition more carefully. The optimum training diet will not make you a Wimbledon champion—unless you've got the shots. However, when training and playing become a serious part of your life, you must meet the special nutritional needs that are created before your tennis skills can be fully developed and showcased.

The training and playing schedules of many elite players set up large energy and carbohydrate requirements. At a lower level of play, carbohydrate needs may not be as great, but may still be beyond the level supplied in the typical Australian diet. See Chapters 1 and 2 for a full account of the optimum training diet.

#### Body-fat levels

Many players, especially females, do not automatically arrive at the body-fat level that does them justice on the court. Being overweight will reduce your speed and stamina, and increase your suffering during hot days on the court. If you need to lose body fat, read Chapter 3 for advice on setting suitable goals and adopting a healthy plan of eating and exercise.

## Fluid intake during matches and training

Tennis is often played in sweltering conditions. Court surface temperatures of 50 degrees Celsius have been reported from centre court during the Australian Open—and some of the concrete outer courts may be even hotter! When matches drag out to three hours or more, and rallies are long and intense, players can amass large sweat losses. To reduce the risk of dehydration and heat injury, players should follow a plan of fluid intake before, during and after matches to keep reasonable pace with sweat losses.

Be aware of your sweat losses during a match, and be especially aggressive on hot and humid days. Keep a supply of cool and refreshing fluids court-side and grab a drink as appropriate—both in terms of your needs as well as opportunities during the match. On some days it may be sufficient to drink between sets, but it is probably good practice to grab a quick drink as you change ends after every second game. After the match, the remaining fluid deficit needs to be replaced—hopefully before the next match—to prevent problems of chronic dehydration.

Don't forget about good hydration practices during training either, particularly if you are out in the heat of the day for long periods. Not only will this look after your training performance, but it will give you the opportunity to practise some match strategies, including your choice of drinks.

While water is adequate to replace fluid losses, there may be additional advantages in providing carbohydrate during long intense matches, especially if you are gradually becoming glycogen-depleted over a long week of tournament matches. Carbohydrate intake during the match may help to boost flagging fuel stores and delay the fatigue of muscle and brain. A sports drink—or alternatively, cordial or diluted fruit juice and soft drinks—may provide carbohydrate and fluid needs simultaneously. Read more in Chapters 4.6 and 4.7.

## Life on the circuit

Elite tennis players can look forward to a life of travelling—around Australia and around the world. While this can be exciting, it can also be stressful. It is often hard to meet nutritional needs in unfamiliar surroundings, especially when time and finances are limited. Read the accounts below for practical advice on travelling nutrition. The first article provides general strategies for life on the run, while the story of Sue further illustrates the problems faced by a touring tennis player.

### Tournament tennis

Tournament tennis is challenging from many nutritional viewpoints. Apart from the considerations of being away from home—even for a weekend tournament—the tournament schedule places great demands on nutritional strategies for recovery, and on a player's flexibility and ingenuity. Not only must a player be committed to looking after fluid and carbohydrate needs between matches, but they must do so without a definite time-table of their day's activities.

Since each day's match draw is determined by the results of the previous day's play, players receive short notice about their daily schedule. Forward planning is also made difficult by the loose nature of the daily timetable. While the starting time for the first match of each session can be set, all other matches simply follow in succession. Given the great range in the duration of matches, it is often difficult for a player to predict accurately the time of their matches.

As in the case of Sue below, tournament players must be learn to be adaptable with their eating plans—having a clear idea of the goals of competition nutrition, but being prepared to handle all possible outcomes in a day's play.

### PROFILE
*The travelling athlete—an accidental tourist*

Take a modern athlete and you have probably also got a seasoned traveller, both within Australia and overseas. At the elite level, frequent international competition is demanded by both the economics and performance standards of many sports. In addition to big events such as World Championships and the Olympic and Commonwealth Games, many top athletes undertake regular training/competition tours overseas, in search of better weather during Southern Hemisphere winters, specialised training such as altitude training, or general fame and fortune on the competition circuit.

National competitions and championships have opened up domestic travelling. In some sports this is no longer an annual national title, but a week-by-week requirement to go on the road. Even recreational-level athletes can be caught up in this mobile world. Who hasn't travelled away to a basketball tournament, triathlon or tennis competition? Some athletes even choose to combine an overseas event with their recreational or business travel—for example, for their annual holiday they might go to New York to run the marathon, or do a triathlon in Fiji.

While travel provides its own rewards and opportunities, for the athlete with special nutritional goals it can also pose some challenges. Some of the food related problems you may face as a travelling athlete are:

- being in a foreign country with a different food supply and different eating customs. As a result, it may be difficult to obtain the types of foods that you like, and that you know will meet your dietary goals. The local food customs may not assist with your nutritional needs as an athlete, and it can be hard to find out the composition of foods and dishes, especially if you don't speak the language. For example, many an athlete with a fussy palate has lost weight because they did not find the local fare to their liking, while others have struggled to find enough carbohydrate sources to load up for an endurance event.

- being unable to prepare your own foods—needing to rely on restaurants and take-aways. Often when you are travelling for short periods you will be staying in a hotel or other accommodation that provides minimal facilities for food preparation or storage. Not only is it expensive to buy all your meals individually, but you are often compromised by the type of food outlets available and the times that you can be served.

- communal eating. So, you are staying in a Games Village or on campus in an institution. You might be lucky enough to be provided with unlimited access to a menu designed for athletes. Foolproof?—unfortunately not. There are many pitfalls to eating in a communal setting, including being mesmerised by the quantities and varieties of food, and being distracted by the eating habits of those around you.

- distraction. Sometimes, just being away from home creates a holiday atmosphere. Indeed for some athletes the trip may actually be doubling as a vacation. As a result, many athletes find that their trips away are sabotaged by a 'let's just enjoy ourselves' spirit.

- travelling itself. Food intake and nutritional goals can become separated when you are actually on the move. Travelling can be stressful, involving long hours, changes in your body clock, and disruption to your training schedule.

It is easy to see how an athlete will not eat—and thus compete or train—at an optimal level under these circumstances.

Eating well as a travelling athlete requires a three-pronged attack:

1 Be clear about your nutritional goals, and how these might change at various times in training and competition. Read through the appropriate sections in Part One of this book.

2 Plan ahead and prepare for your trip. It is often possible to organise food opportunities to suit your needs ahead of time.

3 While you are away, be assertive about handling nutrition decisions to make sure that your nutritional goals are achieved.

HINTS FOR THE TRAVELLING ATHLETE

Prepare ahead
- Find out what to expect at your travel destination(s) and what challenges your training or competition schedule will throw out. Good sources of information are other athletes who have blazed the trail ahead of you, and the organisers of the events you plan to do. Other athletes can usually give you a lengthy account of what to do and what not to do—usually from bitter experience.
- Plan your accommodation with meals in mind. If you are planning to stay in the same place for a long period, or if you have special nutritional needs that may be hard to meet by conventional arrangements (e.g. unusual meal times), then you might be best to find lodgings that provide full cooking facilities. Even facilities for minimal food preparation and storage—e.g. a fridge in your hotel room—can promote better flexibility and possibilities for food intake. Another consideration is to choose an area that is close to shops or restaurants, especially if you will have limited means of transport. For long trips when you are continually on the move, a mobile home or caravan may be an alternative to a succession of hotels.
- Pre-arrange meals where appropriate. Looking over your travel arrangements, you should consider the meals that will be professionally catered—whether by an airline, a restaurant or a hotel. Often it is possible and useful to contact these people ahead of time and arrange to have special meals organised. The hospitality industry does not always do justice to the special needs of athletes. Don't leave yourself open to problems such as inadequate carbo-hydrate intake, excess fat and kilojoules for those with lower energy needs, and nouvelle cuisine for a pack of hungry high-energy consumers. This can also help to reduce waiting time, and make meal times less confusing when travelling with a large group.

  Give the airline or caterers ample notice, and where possible a menu outline. Airlines often have alternative menus, such as 'vegetarian', 'low-fat/high fibre' or 'Pritikin-style', and will be pleased to supply extra bread and fruit for hungry carbohydrate-eaters. It may pay to check what the airline means by its special diet classification—for example, their 'low-fat' diet may simply be a bland diet suitable for someone with gastrointestinal disorders.

- Take a food supply with you. Depending on where you are going and how long you will be away, you may decide to bring some or all of your own food requirements. For example, if you are driving interstate, an Esky may allow you to bring many of your meals or food items for a couple of days. Even if you are travelling overseas for extended times, an emergency food supply can be of great value.

  What you should take will depend on the difficulties that you anticipate with the food supply at your travel destination(s)—for example, whether food items will simply be unavailable there, whether you may not have suitable time and access to go shopping, or whether your travel budget will not spread far. In some Asian and Eastern Bloc countries one or all of these barriers may apply.

  Food items that are sturdy, non-perishable, and require no cooking may be of great value on an overseas trip. See the table on the following page for ideas. These supplies can be supplemented with fresh foods such as bread, fruit, low-fat milk and yoghurts once you have settled in a spot. Keep a food stash for emergencies such as missing a meal, or for times when you need to supplement the meals that have been organised for you. For example, you may come home from a sponsor's dinner at a fancy restaurant feeling that you are still hungry and that your legs will require extra carbohydrate for tomorrow's exercise challenge.

  A low-dose broad-range multivitamin and mineral supplement may be in order if you are unsure of the quality of the food supply or your opportunities to set up a consistent eating pattern.

On the trip: assert yourself
- Look after yourself while actually on the move. Realise that travelling can be extremely boring for an athlete. It may be a time of enforced inactivity (and lower energy needs). Don't equate boredom with hunger and simply eat for entertainment. Eat to a plan, and if you have pre-arranged your meals—e.g. with the airline—stick to this schedule. Watch your fluid balance, especially when flying in pressurised air-cabins. Drink plenty of fruit juices or low-joule drinks, depending on your energy needs. Caffeine drinks (coffee, tea and cola drinks) may dehydrate you if drunk in large quantities, and alcohol is a problem for the same reason.
- Be careful with food safety. 'Traveller's Trots' and 'Delhi Belly' can make a mess of athletic performance. Don't take any risk with food poisoning in foreign countries. Heed the local warnings—you will be told where the water is safe to drink, where it is unwise to eat fresh produce, and which eating places are generally 'safe'.

- Make good choices in restaurants (see Golf Chapter) and with take-aways (see Basketball chapter). These may form a greater part of your diet when travelling than when you are at home.
- Eating well in a cafeteria-style dining hall, commonly part of an athlete's village or university accommodation, can be harder than it looks. Focus on what you need rather than what everybody else is eating (see Swimming chapter).

If you apply the same dietary commitment during your travels as you do while at home, then your trip should reward you with sporting success in addition to new stamps in your passport!

PROFILE: SUE
*Tournament nutrition*

Sue was sure that she knew her nutritional goals for competition, but turning theory into practice in tournament tennis was a difficult task. But she was convinced that it was a crucial part of sustaining her performance level over the week of competition. Too many times she had watched the final being fought out between players she should have beaten, while she had bowed out in dismal style in the middle of the tournament. Often she felt that she had eaten badly over the week and the effects had gradually taken their toll, leaving her tired and unable to play at anywhere near her best.

Of course, it wasn't always just food that caused problems. Life on the circuit often meant lack of sleep, homesickness, and more stress and challenge than was good for her game. It had been especially hard in the early days on the satellite circuit. Not only was the life-style new and bewildering, but conditions were harder for those struggling to make themselves known.

Being short of cash usually meant staying in cheap accommodation away from the tennis centre, and having to spend precious time travelling on public transport to get to and from matches. Access to food, at least the right sort of food, was limited by both time and money and often many days passed before a properly planned meal was managed. In these circumstances it was hard to keep coming up, day after day, particularly if the three or four days of the tournament were preceded by qualifying rounds.

Sue welcomed the improved conditions that accompanied her recent graduation to the Grand Prix circuit. She was now entitled to stay in good hotels situated close to the competition venues, and caterers provided a spread of food in the player facilities at the courts. With food being more accessible, the major challenges now lay in the unpredictable nature of the game of tennis itself.

Sue talked the situation over with a sports dietitian and they agreed that the main principles of tournament nutrition were:

- Maximise and speed-up recovery after each match—particularly long, gruelling battles—by beginning carbohydrate and fluid restoration immediately the match is over. Ideally, start with a carbohydrate snack and/or drink within 15–30 minutes of the end of play.
- When there is a long gap between matches—overnight or a rest day—continue to eat nutritiously, with the emphasis on carbohydrate intake.
- Eat before each match to feel comfortable and refuelled—ideally a light snack about two hours pre-match. Make sure that fluids are topped up on hot days.
- Experiment with a sports drink during matches, drinking to keep pace with fluid losses and carbohydrate needs. Long matches and hot days require extra vigilance.

Separated into its components like this it seemed easy to make a plan. However, Sue explained that difficulties arose because of the loose and unpredictable time-table of events. The day's match schedule was variable, crude and given at short notice. Unless you were drawn for the first match on each court, you could not be sure of the time you were playing. While you could predict an approximate time for the fourth match on court 1, there was never the certainty of a fixed time-table.

This made it difficult to time the pre-match meal or to know what to have between two matches (a singles then a doubles match) on the same day. Sue remembered back to some disastrous experiences, like the occasion when she was scheduled for the third match of the afternoon, and had eaten a reasonable lunch just before the start of the session. Not only was the first match a one-sided affair lasting 35 minutes, but the second match was forfeited after five minutes due to an ankle injury to one of the players. Suddenly, Sue found herself on the court, with a fuller stomach than she would have liked.

On another occasion, during a satellite tournament, Sue had eaten her packed lunch in anticipation of her match, only to find that a rain delay put matches back indefinitely. What was she to do then? Go hungry, or take a chance and eat a snack? And would the little tennis centre kiosk stock anything that passed for high-carbohydrate, low-fat food? Apart from anything else, the worry of making the right decision interfered with her game.

Post-match eating was still sometimes a problem, even with the courtside meals available for the players. When centre court matches stretched into the night, Sue found herself finishing after the caterers had gone home for the day. This left only restaurants (often too late to find one open) or hotel room service (often unsuitable menus). And of course, with late games, sleep sometimes took priority over eating.

The dietitian suggested that two philosophies were needed to handle the situation. First was the idea of flexibility. It would be good to plan the ideal way of tackling a nutritional goal, but it would be better to have a 'plan B' up her sleeve for sudden changes of schedule.

For example, the ideal match preparation would be a light meal about 2–2¹/₂ hours pre-match, followed by a warm-up hit and perhaps a top-up with extra fluids (water) before the match. Matches set to a definite schedule, such as the first match in a session, could be tackled in this fashion.

However, with an uncertain time-table, additional or alternative snacks would be needed at hand. Ready-to-go liquid meal supplements—for example, Exceed Sports Nutrition Supplement—would be particularly versatile in helping to fill in the gaps and handle emergencies. Being liquid and easy to digest, they could supply a nutritious, carbohydrate-based meal without the discomfort of solid food. This would be handy between two matches close together, or as a top-up to an earlier meal when the next match was running late. They could also be a quick no-preparation snack after the game, or a boost to turn a sandwich snack into a more filling meal. With a bit of experimentation, there should be many other food ideas for this trouble-shooting role.

Being self-reliant is the other helpful philosophy. Even at the big tournaments where hotels and court catering are provided, many players choose to organise their own apartments with cooking facilities. This allows them to be more in control, cooking the meals they want at the times they want—although they can fall back on the other food facilities when they want a break. In addition, after weeks on the circuit, it is often nice to have some home cooking rather than restaurant fare. Sometimes, it makes the difference between succumbing to homesickness/travel fatigue or not.

At the lower rungs of the circuit, where the lifestyle isn't so rich and famous, being self-reliant is even more important. If you can afford to stay in a unit, perhaps sharing costs in a group, then with some organisation you may be able to supply the bulk of your own meals. Even in billet or hotel accommodation, you can organise some of your supplies—a travelling food kit can be a great help (see story above and the following table). Having your own food and drinks at the court can be important in making your tournament nutrition happen as planned—again, what you want, when you want it.

Poor nutrition will undoubtedly put your tennis performance below par, through gradual muscle fuel depletion and dehydration in the short-term, and perhaps nutritional deficiencies and weight problems

## NON-PERISHABLE FOOD SUPPLIES FOR THE TRAVELLING ATHLETE

* Liquid meal preparations:  Powder type (e.g. Sustagen) if you need to conserve space

  Liquid ready-to-go types (e.g. Exceed Sports Nutrition Supplement) for times when you do not have food preparation facilities or when the local water supply is unsafe.

* Breakfast cereals and powdered low-fat milk
* Dried fruit, fruit juice packs, and canned fruit (comes in plastic 'snack packs' if you need to save on weight)
* Quick cook noodle and pasta varieties
* Muesli bars and slices (preferably not the chocolate-coated types)
* Dried biscuits or rice cakes with jam or honey

(or Vegemite if you are going to be homesick!)

* Low-dose broad-range multivitamin mineral supplement (if you are unsure of the consistency and the quality of your food intake)

over a long tour. With better planning, not only can you avoid all these physiological traps, but you can go into matches with the confidence boost of knowing you are at your best. There is every chance that you will meet an opponent, even someone with more talent than yourself, who has not prepared for their nutritional needs as well. Your commitment may well mean their loss.

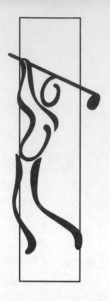

# Golf

Golf is a sport of many levels. At one end of the spectrum are the thousands of Australians who enjoy a social round of nine or eighteen holes on weekends. At the other are some of the highest paid sportspeople in this country—for example, of the top twenty earners in Australian sport for 1990, fourteen were golf players.

Golf is basically a game of skill. A handicapping system operates to level the golfing ability of beginners, and for many recreational players the fun and incentive of golf is not only to play against others but to lower personal handicap scores.

Competitive golf is played at both amateur and professional levels. State and national amateur titles are conducted, with the players involved often struggling to support themselves while practising and playing golf for the requisite hours each day. Golfers can turn professional either through an apprenticeship or by attending Player's School. Under both schemes, potential pro-golfers undertake business studies as well as learning golf skills. While some professional golfers become attached to golf clubs and concentrate on providing golf tuition and running golf shops, others look to making their mark on the professional competitive circuit in Australia, and perhaps overseas.

### Training

Recreational golfers may practise their golf game by simply playing. At the other end of the spectrum, professional competition golfers can spend up to eight hours a day on the golf course, practising specific skills, playing practice rounds or playing in actual competitions. Even during a competition, many players will conduct a practice session at the end of the day's play.

Some players also include general fitness training in their competition preparation—for example, weight training or aerobic activities such as running and swimming. While this training may not directly improve golf skills, some players believe that improved fitness will reduce the deterioration in skills caused by fatigue, and that improved strength may help in the transference of power to the ball.

### Competition

A round of competition golf is played over 18 holes, with golf tournaments being conducted either as a single round on one day, or as multi-day competitions of two or four rounds on consecutive days. In a tournament, there are usually two tee-off times—a morning group starting between 7.00 and 9.00am, and an afternoon group beginning between 11.00am and 1.00pm. A round typically takes three to five hours to play, depending on the skill level of the player and the number of other players on the course. The average golf course is seven kilometres from first to last hole, although a player may walk 10–20 kilometres in a game depending on the accuracy of their shots.

In Australia, winter is the pro-am competition season and professional players typically travel on a circuit between club tournaments. During this season a pro-golfer could play in ten tournaments, for a total of fifteen days of competition, each month. The major international tournaments in Australia are played from January to March and from October to December, flanking the major season overseas. Australian golfers may launch themselves on the international circuit, with either an American or European tour from April to October. The world's best golfers are almost continually on tour, with players such as Greg Norman spending only a few months at home each year.

### Physical characteristics

Golf is a game of skill rather than physical fitness and physical attributes. Therefore top golfers come in many shapes and sizes, with Brett Ogle and Chris Patton showing the extremes among current players. In general, since most players do not undertake intense daily exercise the average body-fat levels of top golfers are higher than aerobically-trained athletes.

**Typical physique (elite Australian Amateur golfers)**

|  | Male | Female |
| --- | --- | --- |
| Height | 175–186cm | 161–168cm |
| Weight | 72–81kg | 58–62kg |
| Skinfolds | 85–118mm | 96–135mm |

### Common nutrition issues

#### Is overweight a handicap?

Players such as American pro-golfer Chris Patton, weighing in at around 140kg, raise the question of whether high body-fat levels affect golf performance. Certainly, being significantly overweight is not an ideal situation in terms of general health. In terms of direct golf skill, we might speculate that a large girth could reduce the flexibility of a player's swing, but equally, that being heavier could provide greater momentum to transfer to the ball.

Theoretically, overweight might also handicap a golfer by reducing general fitness levels and making the player more prone to physical fatigue—and thus more likely to suffer loss of skill and mental concentration. Since body fat works as an insulator, an overweight golfer would also be expected to suffer greater heat intolerance in hot conditions. In both cases, fatigue could cause a drop in skill level over the course of the round and over the days of a tournament.

Of course, these are all theoretical concepts and there is no scientific evidence to support the belief that all overweight players will improve their golfing game by losing body fat. In fact, Craig Stadler, another heavyweight American golfer, reputedly lost body fat only to find that his golf swing was disrupted. To be fair, the blame might equally be placed on his emotional/psychological adjustment to weight loss as well as the direct physical changes.

The best advice is to find a body weight and body-fat level that is healthy and comfortable for you, and to remember that a sport like golf will allow a greater range of tolerance with its ideal physical characteristics. If you do feel that your health and fitness could be improved by loss of body fat, read Chapter 3 for safe and sensible advice to achieve it. By achieving weight loss gradually with a healthy diet and exercise program, you should improve your self-confidence as well as your physical condition. Both effects could be good for your game.

#### Training nutrition

The principles of optimum training nutrition are essentially those of a healthy eating plan, and apply to golfers who play on weekends as well as those who spend eight hours a day on the golf course. Of course as energy expenditure increases with increased training loads, so do requirements for energy and carbohydrate. Read Chapters 1 and 2 for details of the optimum training diet.

#### Tournament nutrition

A top golfer must strive to maintain skills and concentration over three to five hours, perhaps for days on end. Once physical fatigue sets in, deterioration in such skills can be expected. Although a golfer is not faced with the level of strenuous exercise faced by other athletes, prolonged moderate-level activity accompanied by the stress of competition and often inclement weather conditions, can take its toll. Both dehydration and low blood-sugar levels are possible physical hazards to face during competition, and each would be expected to impair golfing performance.

Sweat losses may be considerable when tournaments are played in hot and windy environments or even when high adrenalin levels combine with moderate conditions. Although many golf courses provide drink stations for players, they may be at infrequent intervals and not a significant source of fluid replacement during a game. Since players will usually miss a meal while playing a round, they may be faced with no carbohydrate intake for five or six hours. Combined with exercise and nervous stress, this situation may cause a drop in blood-sugar levels in susceptible individuals, affecting brain function and skill.

When tournaments are held over several days the situation may be compounded, particularly with respect to inadequate fluid replacement. Does your weight drop markedly over the tournament, a sign of chronic dehydration? If you find yourself eating only two meals a day (before and after the day's competition), insufficient kilojoule intake can be another cause of weight loss, and inadequate carbohydrate can add to fatigue levels.

The careful golfer leaves nothing to chance, taking provisions out onto the course to meet the nutritional needs that will arise in competition. There is no need to miss meals or to dehydrate. The plan may vary with individuals and with competition settings, but you should decide for yourself how much fluid you are likely to lose through sweating and how important it is for you to keep up carbohydrate levels during a round. Experiment in practice rounds under simulated competition conditions to determine both your needs and the best way to meet them.

Carbohydrate drinks such as sports drinks, fruit juice and soft drink provide a simple way of consuming fluids and carbohydrates. Work out a schedule of intake that keeps you feeling comfortable. Aim for frequent intake of small amounts—say 150ml every twenty minutes, and keep drinks cool. Food such as sandwiches, fruit or muesli bars can provide additional or alternate forms of carbohydrate intake, and unless you are extremely nervous, these are not likely to cause gastric discomfort. See Chapters 4.6 and 4.7 for more details.

Despite the stress of competition, the golfer should aim to eat well before and after the day's competition. See Chapter 4.4 for discussion about suitable pre-event meals, and be prepared to promote recovery after each round by looking out for fluid and carbohydrate needs as soon as you have finished. This might mean a snack before you go back out onto the practice fairways.

### Life on the circuit

When you are travelling on the golf circuit, both within the country or overseas, meeting your nutritional needs can be a challenge. Whether you are eating in restaurants or catering for yourself, it is often difficult to get what you want at the right time. And to be at your best, both in spirit and in physical form, you need to be on top of your nutrition goals. Read the Tennis chapter for advice about travelling nutrition, and find handy hints for restaurant eating in the guide below.

### Alcohol intake

A golf game traditionally finishes at the 'nineteenth hole'—the bar in the clubrooms. It is also traditional to share a round with your golf partners. Of course this does not necessarily have to mean alcohol intake, but in most cases it probably does.

Read the comments about alcohol in Chapter 1.6. While there may be no harm in having a couple of drinks, it is easy to slip into a pattern of drinking more than you realise or need. It is probably better to avoid alcohol intake during tournaments—after all, you need all the skills and concentration that your brain can muster.

PROFILE
*Waiter—a healthy meal please!*

Most people eat at restaurants occasionally—and for that matter, on special occasions. Under these circumstances it is usual to relax everyday nutritional goals and enjoy a special meal, or even to have a total dietary splurge. However, for athletes on the circuit, continually travelling and relying on hotel accommodation, eating out becomes the way of life.

When restaurants become the major source of your food intake, it is important to know how to make your nutritional requirements turn up on your plate. This is even more crucial when your nutritional requirements are skewed by strenuous exercise—for example, if you are training intensely or competing in heavy competition. In the competition setting, of course, the right food intake is crucial to let you achieve your optimum performance.

The food provided in restaurants generally typifies Australian or Western tastes, and is perhaps a little more exotic than home cooking. Therefore, it can be higher in fat, salt and sugar, and lower in carbohydrate and fibre than the optimum training diet discussed in Chapter 1. This provides an immediate problem in that an athlete may not easily achieve daily carbohydrate requirements. Weight gain may also result because of the temptation to overeat total quantities of food and to over-consume fat in particular.

Of course, it is not always the fault of the restaurant or its food. Many athletes cause their own problems by eating completely out of character—forgetting their nutritional goals and their usual meal patterns. Those who are normally happy with cereal and toast for breakfast suddenly get distracted by the Eggs Benedict on the menu. And three-course hot lunches begin to replace the customary sandwiches and fruit.

Meal timing can also be a problem. Restaurant hours may not always suit your training or competition schedule. You may finish late at night, or need to start early in the morning, and find that you are out of step with the hospitality industry. Even if you appreciate that recovery will be enhanced after a strenuous session by eating carbohydrate immediately, getting those carbohydrates could be another thing. You may find a restaurant open, but then be stymied by the long delay before your order is taken and the food appears in front of you.

And then there is the matter of money. Unless you are a very successful athlete, or the restaurant is included in the circuit hospitality, you may find yourself making food decisions on the basis of financial considerations rather than nutritional concerns.

For general considerations about eating on the circuit, see the Tennis chapter for an account of the travelling athlete. Meanwhile the following hints may help you to cope well with restaurant eating— whether it be a one-off occasion or your everyday life. The table on p. 275 summarises some specific tips for choosing well in particular restaurants, focusing on special tactics to ensure adequate carbohydrate intake, as well as skills to prevent excessive kilojoule intake for those at risk.

## HINTS FOR EATING WELL IN A RESTAURANT

- Set nutritional goals for a restaurant meal, according to its importance in the overall scheme of your performance. If it is a special or unusual occasion you may decide to take a more relaxed attitude. However if this is a crucial time in training or competition, or eating out is your way of life, then choose food for its nutritional contribution rather than its taste appeal alone.

- It helps to be familiar with a restaurant. If you are in an unfamiliar area, ask advice—especially from other athletes.

  When you travel to a new place, scout around to see what restaurants are available. Being armed with some knowledge lets you plan in advance where you will eat. If you wait until you are tired and desperately hungry to look or decide on a place, you will probably make a compromised decision. Also, remember that many restaurants are run as a franchise or chain—if you find a good place in one city, you may be able to make use of its equivalents on your travels.

- Remember that restaurants are a hospitality industry, and by rights should be pleased to provide the service that you request. Don't be afraid to arrange for your special needs—whether it be meal timing, or the type of food you would like.

- There may be occasions when it is important to eat straight away, to promote rapid recovery or to conserve precious sleep time. To avoid long waits in a restaurant, try 'phoning the restaurant ahead of time and organise your order. This can be especially useful if you are in a large group.

- Smorgasbord restaurants generally offer a speedier service, plus more freedom of choice over what you eat. However, you may need to use greater skills to avoid the distraction of quantities and types of food that are not on your menu.

- If saving money is a priority, you may be able to make up your own breakfast and lunch meals from easy-to-prepare foods that you can buy or keep in your room. Make the most of dinner in a restaurant to maintain variety and make up for any nutritional shortfalls in the other meals. (Of course, depending on your schedule, you may like to make lunch the main meal of the day.)

# HOW TO MEET YOUR NUTRITIONAL GOALS IN A RESTAURANT

| Situation | Tips to increase carbohydrate intake | Tips to avoid excess kilojoule intake |
| --- | --- | --- |
| General comments | Be aware that you will be working against the Western trend to eat protein (and fat) with carbohydrate foods as an accompaniment. Either choose a dish that is based on carbohydrate, or order a smaller serve of a protein based meal (meat, fish, chicken, egg, cheese, etc.), and add generous side-serves of carbohydrate foods (fruit/juice, bread, potato, rice, noodles, etc.) | Choose only as much as you need—limit the number of courses or ask for smaller serves. If all else fails, leave what you don't require. Be vigilant about limiting fat intake, and watch the added extras with meals—e.g. garlic bread, french fries, and high-kilojoule drinks (alcohol especially). Look for bulky low-joule foods or low-joule drinks to fill up with instead. Take extra care with buffet or smorgasbord type meals, especially with regard to coming back for seconds. |
| Breakfast | Breakfast is perhaps the easiest meal to cater for. Nutritious carbohydrate foods include juice, fruit, cereals, toast, muffins and crumpets. If you would like something warm try porridge, pancakes, baked beans or spaghetti. | Limit fat intake by asking for low-fat milk on your cereal and by being a miser with the butter/margarine on breads. Your main enemies are croissants, and high-fat cooked meals such as bacon and eggs. |
| Lunch | Meals based on breads—rolls or sandwiches—are quick and nutritious. Have a | Watch the spreads on your bread and oily dressings. Otherwise, fill up the meal with |

| Situation | Tips to increases carbohydrate intake | Tips to avoid excess kilojoule intake |
|---|---|---|
| | thick layer of bread and fill with a little protein and lots of salad. Other variations include hearty soups with bread, baked potatoes with a filling, and gourmet hamburgers. If you need extra kilojoules, finish up with scones, muffins or a healthy cake. Fruit and fruit salad, and low-fat icecream or yoghurt are other high-carbohydrate foods. Drinks include juices, soft drinks and sports drinks—or if you really need to push the kilojoules and carbohydrates, ask for a low-fat fruit smoothie. | salads. Low-joule drinks include iced water (ask for a jug), plain mineral water and diet soft drinks. You may be able to afford a dessert, but save 'fat' kilojoules by removing cream or cream cheese icing. What about a low-fat yoghurt, or a soft-serve of the same? Vitari is another low-fat 'icecream'. Fruit is always a good choice. |
| General restaurant/ French restaurant | The usual choice of an entree and main course based on protein foods blocks out room for the carbos. If you need an entree, try thick vegie soup with bread. For a main course, choose a main or entree-size protein meal (consider it a side-dish) and order extra serves of potatoes, rice or noodles as well as your vegies. Stick to non-fat | Apart from the total quantity of food you eat (see general comments above), your main concern is your fat intake. Choose lean cuts of meat/fish/chicken (e.g. avoid processed meats, fatty mince meats and high-fat duck). Ask for non-fat cooking methods—grilling, stewing, dry baking. A large baked potato has plenty of carbos for less |

| Situation | Tips to increase carbohydrate intake | Tips to avoid excess kilojoule intake |
|---|---|---|
| | cooking methods (see next column). High-carbohydrate, low-fat desserts include fruit salad, low-fat icecreams, sorbets and yoghurts, rice pudding and fruit crumble. Bread and high-carbohydrate drinks (see lunch ideas) can also boost total carbohydrate intake. | kilojoules than small roast potatoes or chips. Watch sauces and gravies that are based on butter or cream, or oil and butter brushed on your vegies. Don't hesitate to request that your meal is served without the sauces, or with the sauces on the side (to use sparingly). Ask for plain bread rather than oily herb or garlic breads, and for salads that are left plain or with low-oil dressings. You can decide to go without dessert all together or perhaps share one with someone else. If you would like something sweet try some fruit, a little low-fat icecream/ yoghurt/sorbet—or perhaps a single chocolate with your tea/coffee. |
| Italian | Pasta is a great carbohydrate food, but be aware that many pasta dishes are not what they seem. Lasagnes and cannelloni, for example, may be more filling than pasta, and the fillings may be high in fat—oil, fatty meat | Order an entree course of pasta for your main meal and be extra careful to choose a low-fat sauce—even if that means making a special request. If the sauce arrives in greater quantities or with more oil than you expected, try to eat only a little |

| Situation | Tips to increase carbohydrate intake | Tips to avoid excess kilojoule intake |
|---|---|---|
| | and cheese. High-fat sauces based on cream and oil can also make a spaghetti dish high in fat rather than carbohydrate. Order well—a vegetable or tomato-based sauce is usually best. Meat, chicken and bolognaise sauces can be fine, if the meat is lean and oil is used sparingly. See general restaurant comments for other ideas. | to make the pasta tasty. |
| Chinese Malaysian Thai | Rice and noodles are the Malaysian mainstay of Asian cuisine. Your best bet is to order stirfried meat and vegetable dishes, adding these as a topping to bowls of steamed rice or noodles. Watch the traps that add lots of fat to a meal so that you can concentrate on the carbohydrates. (see next column) | Since most dishes are based on small amounts of meat/fish/chicken, most of the fat in Asian cooking comes from oil added in cooking. Avoid dishes that have been battered or deep fried, and request that stirfries are cooked with minimum oil. Base meals on plain rice or noodles rather than special fried rices— there is already plenty of flavour in the dishes you will add to the rice/ noodle base. Avoid banquets with numerous courses and lots of spring rolls and deep-fried finger-foods. If you are sharing courses in a group, make a conscious decision about what |

| Situation | Tips to increase carbohydrate intake | Tips to avoid excess kilojoule intake |
| --- | --- | --- |
| | | you will eat—e.g. how many times you will fill up your bowl. It is tempting to keep picking, and refilling your bowl, without judging how much you have eaten. |
| Indian | As for Chinese above— use steamed rice as a base for the rest of the meal. Other good carbohydrate foods are lentils, chickpeas, and Indian bread— preferably the non-fried varieties. | As for Chinese, ask for dishes cooked with little oil, and avoid fried and battered foods, including samosas and fried breads. Small serves of curries eaten on rice can be a great meal—but make sure that you quench your thirst with low-joule drinks after a hot spicy meal! |
| Mexican | Rice, beans and Mexican flat bread (tortillas) are all good carbohydrate foods. Try not to fill up on too much cheese, meat and sour cream—you may not have enough room for the foods you really need. In some ways it can help to order individual items from the menu rather than set main courses. You can put together some tostadas, beans, rice and extra tortillas, for example, rather than a plate full of high-fat items. | Be wary of the giant main courses that are legendary in Mexican restaurants and of the high-fat dishes. As suggested in the Carbohydrate column, you may be better to order à-la-carte to choose just what you need. Corn chips are made with oil and are therefore high in kilojoules, so it is a mistake to sit with a pile of nachos smothered in cheese and sour cream in front of you. |

| | |
|---|---|
| Pritikin and health restaurants | Many restaurants now cater for high-carbohydrate low-fat meals. Be a little wary of restaurants labelled 'health food'—there may still be plenty of high-fat ingredients used, such as pastry, oil and cheese. Nevertheless, many restaurants meet the challenge well, providing dishes that meet the guidelines for healthy nutrition as well as appealing to gourmet tastebuds. If you need to watch your kilojoule intake, be careful about the total quantity that you eat—it is still possible to eat too much of a good thing. |
| Alcohol | Most people associate restaurants with 'wining and dining', and a couple of glasses of alcohol can be a pleasant part of a healthy meal and an enjoyable night. However, think carefully about the effect of alcohol on your performance. You may decide to forego alcohol when dining out in the midst of competition or strenuous training, or leave it for special occasions rather than every time you eat in a restaurant. |

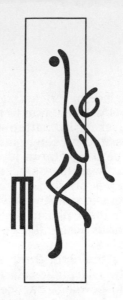

# Cricket

Cricket is a game of skill and tradition that touches the lives of most Australians each summer. Teams of eleven play against each other, with slightly different rules governing the limited-over (one-day) games compared to those based on two innings for each side (four or five day games). While both men's and women's competitions exist, it is the men's scene that dominates with lucrative professional and international competition. It is hard to progress though the ranks of district and state (Sheffield Shield) level cricket to this level. Most cricket in Australia is played at a social and recreational level with many leagues and competitions carrying grades down to 'F' level.

Roughly speaking, a cricket team is broken into specialist batsmen, specialist bowlers and a wicket-keeper. Theoretically, all team members get to bat and to field, while usually only the specialists are required to undertake the task of bowling. The game is based on skill, and only at a high level of play and only in recent years, has there been a requirement for reasonable aerobic fitness. Even so, there are many top-level cricketers who are better titled as sportsmen rather than athletes, and whose off-field activities create as many stories and legends as their on-field exploits.

### Training

Cricket is a summer sport, with the season beginning at the end of October and progressing through to a final series in March–April. At the top level, some cricketers play all year round, travelling to

England to play in their county cricket season. Alternatively, a few cricketers at the top level will continue to train, or at least to remain fit, over winter. However, the usual pattern is to stop playing once the season is over, and unless the cricketer gets involved in another sport over winter—perhaps football—fitness levels may be very poor by the beginning of the next season.

At first-grade cricket level, pre-season training begins around June, most often in the form of general fitness work, and is often unsupervised or left to the individual player. As the season draws closer, organised team training takes over and the component of skills practice is increased.

During the season at a top club, three team training sessions are organised each week between matches. Each session lasts 2–2$^1$/$_2$ hours and involves batting and bowling practice, fielding skills and drills, and perhaps some general running or fitness work. Some individual players at the top level may be motivated to organise their own fitness program in addition to this, and may undertake additional aerobic training and perhaps weights.

In low-grade competition there may be little or no organised training.


### Competition

District cricket is played on weekends with many grades or levels of competition. This may be in the form of two-day fixtures and/or limited over (one-day) competition, with these competitions often happening simultaneously. The state-level cricket competition (Sheffield Shield) is organised into four-day matches (Friday to Monday) and often interrupts the district level season for those who are chosen to play.

Summer is a busy time for international cricket in Australia. The program usually includes a test series (five-day matches) and a World Series Cup (one-day, limited-over matches) played against touring teams from other cricket-playing nations. Between matches, the cricketers may go back to their state level competition, and may train with their state teams or district clubs. When an overseas tour is organised, the Australian team will travel together for a period of time, and may include team training sessions between matches.

The physical requirements of a cricket game vary with the format of the match (multi-day versus limited-over game), and with the player's position in the team. Test games are played at 'gentleman's hours'—six hours of match play plus breaks, between 11.00am and 6.00pm. The limited-over series may also involve day–night matches and a slightly different time-table of play.

Games played in the middle to end of summer are often played in very hot conditions, requiring players to stand for many hours in the sun. Those at most risk of heat stress are those standing out the longest (e.g. the fielding team) and the fast bowlers who may work intensely in short spells over the day. Batsmen who stay in for a long innings may also have to run repeatedly in this heat.

### Physical characteristics

Cricketers come in all shapes and sizes—even at the top level. It has only been in recent years that cricket coaches have demanded that body fat be kept at a reasonable level to accompany the increased fitness level expected of players. A healthier level of body fat would theoretically improve speed, stamina and heat tolerance. Speed becomes important at a high level of play, particularly in the limited-over matches, since skilled fielding and running between wickets is helpful for success. Many fast bowlers have been singled out as deserving of lower body-fat levels and improved fitness, in the belief that this will improve their speed and therefore their delivery, as well as increasing their stamina to bowl and field over the day. Wicket-keepers must be strong as well as agile—in an average day of keeping, the equivalent of 600 squats may be done.

### Common nutrition issues

#### Body-fat levels

If you feel that your life would be healthier, your cricket game faster, and your captain happier by shedding some weight, then opt for a fat-loss program that is based on sensible and long-term principles. Many male (and female) cricketers find themselves wanting to lose weight but not knowing how to do it—nutrition and fitness may never have been a big consideration in their lives. The cricketing lifestyle may not help the cause either, being made up of low-exercise levels, and too much of the good life. Read the account of Duncan below, and Chapter 3 for ideas on healthy fat loss.

#### Training nutrition

Cricketers are among the last group of sportspeople to warm to the idea of a healthy nutrition lifestyle. For most, the rewards will be improved health and vitality, and better weight control. However, for the new breed of cricketers who undertake an organised fitness and training schedule, the special dietary needs of daily training will be met by these same nutrition principles. Read Chapters 1 and 2 for an outline of the optimum diet for health and training.

#### Match day nutrition

Match day nutrition is run on tradition rather than science, even at the top level. Players may rise late, especially if there was a celebration the night before (see the comments on alcohol below), and pre-event meals are variable in quantity and type. Test players staying in hotels may even start the day with a hearty (high-fat) cooked breakfast.

Matches are generally played with a drink break every hour, and a set break for lunch (40 minutes) and tea (20 minutes). A meal is usually eaten in the lunch break, and great tradition prevails in its organisation. At elite-level cricket, meals are catered by the ground social club and can range from a light snack to a heavy meal of roast or fried fish. The legendary 'cricketer's salad' generally consists of cold meats, salads and bread, but may also be high in fat (due to the dressings, added margarine and processed meats) and relatively low in carbohydrate.

Further down the competition scale, the tradition of a 'social' lunch also applies, with the home team responsible for providing the food. Wives and girlfriends may organise a roster or organise for everyone to bring a plate. The time-table varies a little with the schedule of one-day matches, but the tradition remains essentially the same.

After reading Chapter 4, you will see that very few of the state-of-the-art competition nutrition ideas have found their way into cricket. And indeed, it might be argued that with a game of skill, there is less need for such scientific concerns. Nevertheless, cricketers might consider updating some of their competition practices. In terms of comfort and topping up carbohydrate stores, light, high-carbohydrate meals would be more appropriate as pre-match and lunch-time meals.

Combating dehydration is an important issue, and cricketers should drink at least 250–500ml of fluid at each drink break to replace sweat losses on hot days. For those players who are actually working—the batsmen, bowlers and wicket-keeper—the provision of carbohydrate in these drinks may be of additional benefit. Experiment with cordial or a sports drink. Lastly, post-match strategies should promote recovery, especially when in the midst of a multi-day match. Recovery practices include fluid, carbohydrate and rest—not always a priority of cricketers (see comments on alcohol).

### Alcohol intake

Alcohol intake is heavily interwoven in the cricketer's lifestyle. Cricketing traditions include having a beer with the opposition team at the end of the day, or in the case of international cricket (where team tactics frown on being too friendly with the competition) having a beer with your own team-mates. Even during a multi-day match and even at high levels of play, it is acceptable behaviour to go out wining and dining, or drinking and dancing until late into the night. And of course, when the match is over, or the test series has been decided, newspapers often carry a picture of the winning team in their locker rooms celebrating with some victory drinks.

Not only is alcohol intake an expected part of the game, but heavy drinking is also glorified and becomes the stuff of legends. Not only do cricketing afficionados know how many half-centuries were made by an international cricketer on a tour of England, but also the number of cans of beer he drank on the flight home.

Clearly such drinking practices go against the principles of healthy nutrition and optimum performance. Read Chapter 1.6 for a discussion of the role of alcohol in sport. As in other male-dominated team sports, it will take time and a change of attitude before healthier practices become widespread in cricket. It is hoped that the emerging group of first-class cricketers will include sensible drinking practices among their ideas of professionalism—not only looking after their own lives and sporting careers, but providing a role model for thousands of young cricket players.

### Travelling on tour or abroad

Cricketers on tour live out of hotels and suitcases, and in the case of many overseas tours, they may be constantly on the move for a number of months. Standing in the way of optimum nutrition are the usual problems associated with being a travelling athlete, as well as the strong traditions associated with being a cricketer on tour. Remind yourself of your nutrition priorities (Chapters 1 and 2), and for specific advice on travelling nutrition read the sections in the Tennis chapter (the travelling athlete) and the Golf chapter (eating in restaurants).

PROFILE: DUNCAN
*Lose weight or lose match payments!*

There was a new order in at Duncan's cricket club and Duncan was worried. Duncan was a fast bowler, with the potential to be a very fast bowler if he wasn't so fat. The new captain-coach called the team together at the beginning of pre-season training and explained his ideas for a new, fit team that would blast the opposition with speed and professionalism as well as skill. Each player was interviewed separately, and Duncan was given instructions to lose nine kilos—or face fines. A fitness program was drawn up and an appointment set in a fortnight for Duncan to report in on his progress with the weight loss.

Duncan had heard talk like this before. Last year they had told him to lose weight also—the same old nine kilograms. But Duncan had dodged his way though the season, laughing to the club officials that he had carefully developed a life of 'organised sloth'. The weight had stayed put, but his season's figures were moderately successful so no-one had really bothered to pursue the matter.

This year was different, however. The new captain-coach didn't look like he would stand any nonsense, and a new fast-bowler had been recruited. If Duncan wanted to hold his position, it looked like he would have to make some changes. How could he lose the weight?

Duncan tried the 'Israeli Army diet', and after a week achieved nothing except a dislike for green apples. One of his mates told him about the 'Drinking Man's diet'. This sounded like his kind of diet, but they were unable to find a copy. Duncan attended his first fortnightly weigh-in with the captain-coach and found himself fined $200 dollars for the lack of progress. That really hurt! However, the coach then explained that the money would be used to pay for a series of consultations with a sports dietitian.

Duncan was surprised when the dietitian didn't immediately give him a diet sheet. However, she explained that rigid dietary plans were usually only successful in the short-term. If Duncan wanted to go to the trouble of losing weight, he might as well do it properly and lose it forever—by learning a new, healthier lifestyle. The dietitian likened this to the help that he received from the specialist bowling coach at the club. This coach carefully examined Duncan's bowling style, picking out the faults and weaknesses and helping him to remodel and improve his deliveries.

Duncan's typical daily diet was discussed and assessed. The dietitian learned that he lived at home, but was rarely there to eat meals. Nevertheless, it was a potential source of food, and Duncan explained that his mother had become pretty careful about her cooking since his father's heart attack, four years ago. The typical intake for his day is summarised in the table on the following page.

The dietitian was honest in her assessment, telling Duncan that his diet was high in fat and that his alcohol intake was inconsistent with a trim waistline and good performance. The uneven spread of energy over the day—skipped meals and heavy intake late at night—also worked against his weight control. She explained the principles of healthy training nutrition to him (see Chapter 1) and together they negotiated an eating plan that fitted this mould.

Important changes included:

- no more skipping breakfast. With less late nights, Duncan would aim to get up in plenty of time for a healthy breakfast before work.
- a sandwich-based lunch to replace high-fat take-aways. Duncan wasn't too keen on eating fruit, but liked the look of the fresh fruit salad in the shop next to work.
- either a better chosen (low-fat) restaurant meal, or home to some of Mum's healthy cooking. Some serving sizes were given.
- instead of calling out for pizza on late training nights, the dietitian gave Duncan a recipe for a quick, low-fat version, using low-fat cheese and vegetables on pita bread.

**Duncan's diet—before and after**

| | Original diet—a typical day | Healthy weight loss diet—a new daily plan |
|---|---|---|
| Breakfast | none (late for work) | bowl of wholegrain cereal with low fat milk, fruit juice |
| Lunch | pies/sausage rolls, flavoured milk<br>1/week: counter lunch with 2–3 beers | salad sandwich with cheese/ham/chicken/tuna/beef<br>medium serve of fresh fruit salad |
| After training | two or three times/week: 4–5 beers at the pub | 2 light beers (2 per cent alcohol) |
| Dinner | fried fish, chips, salad at the pub | Restaurant or home meal:<br>grilled meat/fish/chicken, medium serve, all fat trimmed.<br>2 bread rolls or large potato, or cup rice/pasta<br>pizza made on large pita bread base with reduced-fat cheese, tomato paste, vegetables, and perhaps diced meat/chicken/seafood. 1 stubbie of light beer or Diet Coke. |
| Later in night | corn chips and Coke while watching TV, or a medium pizza with the lot plus a litre of Coke or couple of stubbies | TV snacks—homemade popcorn (minimum oil), Diet Coke |

- switching to light alcohol beer—and rationing himself to one stubbie a night. Duncan was a bit reluctant, but realised that many of his mates were already moving to this trend because of drink-driving laws.
- replacing Coke with low-joule drinks.

When the plans were laid out side-by-side, Duncan was surprised to see how much food he could now eat. The dietitian assured him that the new diet contained far less kilojoules and far more carbohydrate and vitamins/minerals than his old diet. He tackled the new plan with gusto, and with his fitness program and new attitude felt a new man. Duncan's success exceeded even his own expectations. The weight was lost within two months, and a month later Duncan reached what he considered his new 'fighting weight'. Being fit and motivated, his game became more aggressive and confident. Not only did he keep his place at the club, but he was recently selected to train with the state side.

# Index